A Light in the Darkness

*Transcending Chronic Illness through
the Power of Art and Attitude*

Lisa A. Sniderman

Crimson Cloak Publishing

Cover design by Charlie Aspinall

Printed in the United States of America

ISBN 13: 978-1-68160-557-9

ISBN 10: 1-68160-557-0

For information contact:
Crimson Cloak Publishing
P.O Box 36 Pilot Knob
Missouri 63663

Publisher's Publication in Data

Sniderman, Lisa A.

A Light in the Darkness

1 Non-Fiction 2 Inspirational 3 Biography

Dedication

To my hero of a husband, David, without whose love and support this book would never have been written.

And for Amberlin and all who suffer with chronic illness.

"May you use this illness as a lantern to illuminate the new qualities that will emerge in you."

—John O'Donohue, An Abundance of Blessings

Praise for *A Light in the Darkness*

"Chronic illness challenges us in so many ways, but need not define who we are and what we have to offer. Sniderman is an inspiration. Her memoir provides an honest window into the power of the human spirit through real life examples and wisdom to reimagine what is possible."

— Keith W. L. Rafal, MD, MPH, Founder of Our Heart Speaks, www.ourheartspeaks.org

"Caring for a son with Juvenile dermatomyositis, I was overcome with the truth and rawness (and tears) of Sniderman's moving story. Her words are uplifting, compelling, engaging, and illuminating for anyone living with chronic illness and for those who love them."

— Shannon Malloy, Cure JM Foundation

"Lisa Sniderman is an amazing example of finding unbeatable strength through one's creativity. She inspires others with her passion for her music and art and using them to rise above the incredible challenges of her chronic illness. Bravo!"

— Angelo "Scrote" Bundini, producer and artist

"Sniderman shares valuable wisdom in her open and honest account about overcoming the adversity of living with a chronic illness. A truly inspirational story of the healing power of music and creativity and finding your true purpose."

— Tom Willner, cancer survivor and author of *Having A Ball At Thirty*

"Much like her experience in the MRI scanner, Sniderman treats every 'pulse' she hears and feels in her life as if it were music — understanding that the artistic beauty of life's journey is its individuality and desperate plea to ignore the confinement of having an itinerary."

— David Fiorentino MD, PhD, Professor of Dermatology, Stanford University School of Medicine

"Sniderman's inspirational tale serves to reminds us of what is possible no matter what we are going through in our own lives. Music and art are often powerful healers that provide the hope medicine needed to keep us moving forward each day."

— Vincent James and Joann Pierdomenico, authors of *88+ Ways Music Can Change Your Life* and Founders of Keep Music Alive

"A personal and poignant meditation on healing and hope. Sniderman's brilliant account will surely enlarge empathy, so that more can understand what it means to live with and triumph over struggles."

— Kabir Sehgal, *New York Times and Wall Street Journal* bestselling author and Grammy Award winner

"As a former psychological counselor, poet, and mother of a child with Juvenile Myositis, I am thrilled by Lisa's book. Her story of both living with a chronic illness and finding ways to harness and express her talents to encourage and inspire others is a gift. I know many kids and adults will not only resonate with her story but will be uplifted by it and will find ways to let 'their lights shine' too. This is an important and necessary story, not just for people with Dermatomyositis, but for anyone who struggles with, or loves someone with a chronic illness."

— Suzanne Edison, MA, MFA, Cure JM Board of Directors

"Sniderman's ability to overcome impossible obstacles is nothing short of miraculous. Her positive outlook on life and remarkable passion for the arts has truly helped in her recovery. I highly recommend reading *A Light in the Darkness*. You will find it to be a transformative experience."

— Tim Battersby, Grammy nominee and novelist

"Lisa Sniderman's inspiring life lessons portray the story of struggle, relentless determination and perseverance, leading to her success lifting herself up. Her artistic life is an inspiration to others and an encouraging testament to never giving up in this beautiful universe to make the best out of this life despite challenges."

— Rupam Sarmah, Music Director, composer and filmmaker

"Lisa shares her journey with honesty and grace. The heartfelt ideas and suggestions she offers are useful, inspiring and uplifting — for people dealing with chronic illness or any other life challenge."

— Sarah Moran, health writer and author of the *Take Care* wellness book series

"In this honest and inspiring account of perseverance and triumph, Lisa Sniderman shares her honest insights and encouraging life lessons that you can use to manage the impact of your chronic illness, reignite your lost inspirations and still follow your dreams."

— Tony J. Selimi, Human Behaviour Specialist and international best-selling author of *A Path to Wisdom*

"This is a story of adaptation, of being handed terrible circumstances and finding ways to still follow your dreams and live life on your terms. A well-written book that plunges the reader into the life of someone with a chronic illness, Sniderman shares her journey and the transformation that allowed her to accept her limitations and embrace life as it is, while being a guiding light for others."

— Corrina Thurston, wildlife artist and author

Contents

What You Got

What-what you got
What-what you got

When life is hurling lemons at your face
When you're an old rat and can't race
And you've just lost your mate to that obnoxious tramp
And doors are slamming

When all-all you can do
Is hide till it's through

You got to do what you can with what you got
You gotta move to the groove with what you got
You got to go-o-o-o with the flow—just take it slow
And do what you can with what you got
What-what you got

When all you see are stacks of bills to pay
When you can't get out of bed today
And you've been told 30 days is all you get
And you just put down your cat

When all-all you can do
Is cry till it's through

You got to do what you can with what you got
You gotta move to the groove with what you got
You got to go-o-o-o with the flow—just take it slow
And do what you can with what you got

Whether you like it
Or like it not
Whether he loves you
Or loves you not
It's what-what you got
What-what you got

When you no longer fit inside your jeans
When mom is a total drama queen
And you're watchin' someone else live your dreams
While tv's your family

When all-all you can do
Is bre-ak in two

You got to do what you can with what you got
You gotta move to the groove with what you got
You got to go-o-o-o with the flow—just take it slow
And do what you can with what you got

You got to do what you can with what you got
You gotta move to the groove with what you got
You got to go-o-o-o with the flow—just take it slow
And do what you can with what you got
Don't try to be something that you're not
Just go-o-o-o-o-o with what you got
What-what you got

Prologue
A Gift in Disguise

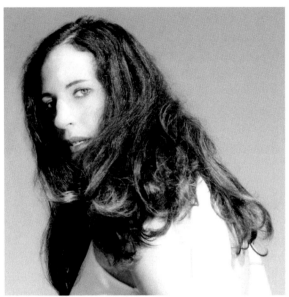

Aoede 2007—Credit Liz Caruana Photography

I remember the first time it hit me that my dream was changing. My husband, David, and I went to Los Angeles for a music workshop in June 2009. We came away crazy excited because we and some of our fine colleagues were offered the opportunity to perform at Caesars Palace in Las Vegas the following year. It was sort of an experiment to prove to the bookers that all of us unsigned indie singer-songwriters, artists, and bands were just as good, if not better, than the acts typically booked in Las Vegas venues. It was our chance to get in front of mega-music-industry professionals and network, network, network. If nothing more than playing at Caesars Palace came of it, I still would have jumped at the opportunity.

But as performance time approached in 2010, I wasn't able to get out of bed or the house, let alone the state. When I made the call to cancel my performance, a dream died.

Never could I have imagined how my life would change when about a year earlier, in April 2008, I was at the dermatologist's office being diagnosed with a rare, chronic autoimmune disease, which, if left untreated, I later learned, could leave me completely debilitated. I had never been limited in doing anything I set my mind and heart to. That's just me. I've always dreamed, believed, and gone for it—whatever "it" was at the moment.

Sometimes "it" would manifest very differently from what I originally envisioned, like the first and only time I attempted hang gliding when I was seventeen or eighteen and nose-dived right off the cliff, scraping my foot because I'd been foolish enough to wear open-toed sandals! Or spending six weeks working an archaeological dig with the Summer Institute of Israel after my senior year in high school, only to end up being one of two in our group who got dehydrated while riding a camel in the desert and had to be given IV fluids at an army base while everyone else waited on the bus. Or that time in college when I took a painting class without any prior drawing experience and was asked to paint a model who was sitting on a chair, which was sitting on a platform. My model's chair, if you could call it that, looked as if it were trying to walk off the platform. Two of its legs were dangling off the edge, along with my model's legs. The model had no form, and her neck and body were so elongated that my art teacher said, "Hey, you should check out Modigliani." I know it was meant as encouragement, but I realized I had no aptitude for perspective and spatial orientation, and without serious training, I wasn't going to go far as an artist.

Nevertheless, I dreamed up a big musical adventure, getting my start as a lead singer in the cover band *Tuesday's Alibi* after my first husband and I divorced in 2002. It was one of those "I'm free! I'll find and reinvent myself" seasons. Of course, when you're young, or young at heart, *and* have your health, you can do anything. Or at least you think you can, so there really isn't much difference.

Did I know anything about the technical aspects of singing? Had I played guitar? Did I write songs? No. I hadn't sung in public since my high school musical *Grease*. I had never touched a guitar. I had played violin in fourth grade and sax in fifth or sixth, but neither of those stuck. I sang as a kid and in high school productions but never landed the coveted lead roles. I had written poems and snippets of lyrics and journal entries for years … but songs?

Between 2002 and 2009, I went after music training with my usual enthusiasm and drive: vocal lessons, guitar lessons, and eventually, songwriting classes and private mentoring. My first attempts were feeble, to say the least. There was homework and endless practice. But I never doubted that I could do it. I never questioned whether to put my expression out there into the Universe. *Tuesday's Alibi* even started playing some of my original songs between 2003 and 2005. I was just starting to discover that I had a muse.

In 2006, I took on the musical identity of Aoede, the Muse of Song. Why Aoede (pronounced "ay-ee-dee")? In Greek mythology, way before the nine celebrated muses, there was a muse of song by that name. In the early 2000s, when my muse flowed and took the form of my songs, I wanted to be affiliated with the ancient muse as a reminder to continually inspire others and be inspired. Aoede launched me on my musical path as a singer-songwriter. Little did I know that years later, the theme of muse would be so central to my life's path and purpose.

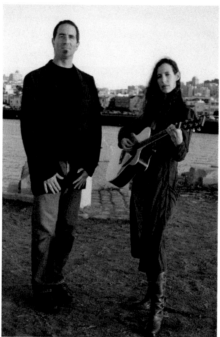

Aoede Nov 2006 with David Sands
Credit Liz Caruana Photography

Like many of you, I had my share of minor health issues during my life prior to being diagnosed with a chronic illness: colds that always turned into crappy, lingering bronchitis, respiratory problems, asthma, and various other ailments. The difference was I could manage them. I used an inhaler. I took antibiotics. I knew I would be miserable for a time and might have to take a few weeks out of life while my body fought to recover. Occasionally I even had to go to the hospital for breathing treatments, but I always recovered. I went back to work. I resumed my life and activities. Although being sick was an inconvenience, I could rest assured that whatever it was would pass.

But chronic illness doesn't pass. That's why it's called *chronic*. You can sit around and wait all you want, but it doesn't get better. I think I was in denial for the first few years after being diagnosed, even though my body was giving me clear signals that something—or multiple things inside me—was diseased. I had always managed before, so I adopted a this-too-shall-pass attitude.

But it never did pass. While my friends and family talked excitedly about their travels, jobs, adventures, shows, tours, weddings, and new babies, I rooted them on but watched from the sidelines, as if viewing a movie I was no longer playing a part in.

What can you do if you have an illness or disability that doesn't go away? You can ignore it. You can live in fear of it. You can fight it and get angry about it. You can scream at it and demand to know why it's there. (If you get a response, do let me know!) You can acknowledge it. You can make friends with it. You can accept it. This process feels similar to the classic stages of grief. I've experienced all the stages on some level, and cyclically—never in tidy chronological order. I go back and forth all the time. When I'm deeply involved in my art or music, or something else that excites me, I often ignore the signals my body is giving me, pretending that my eyes aren't fighting sleep or that my body doesn't desperately need to rest. If my mind is so active and willing and ready to go, go, go, then why should my body stand in the way?

Former NFL coach Ray Rhodes wrote, "At one time, you think you're invincible. This [chronic illness] just can't happen to you, but when it happens, the reality sets in that you either change or you die. You realize you've got only one life." Some days I feel as if I haven't yet made peace with my limitations, with the hard and indisputable fact that I'm no longer invincible. Accepting my new normal in terms of stamina and a radically changed lifestyle has been harder even than accepting I have a chronic disease. But I'd much rather live my life than sit around waiting for it to happen. If this is the life I have now, then I had better make the best of it. I can't, and don't, ask why I have this autoimmune disease; I only ask what I can learn from it and what I can teach. I've embraced the African proverb, "When the music changes, so does the dance."

When life throws you curveballs, it's tempting to give up—on a dream, on a project, on finishing a song. And if you live with a disease or disability, it's easy to succumb to discouragement, self-pity, or even despair. But dreams and significant health challenges aren't mutually exclusive. I'm a living example. It's still possible to find reasons not to give up.

I've overcome many obstacles in pursuit of my dreams. The worst for me was a flare-up of my illness in 2010 that put me in the hospital and rehab for twenty-four days and required several more months of grueling rehab after I returned home to regain my strength and independence. Hope has always been, and will continue to be, my guiding light. It has been central to the life I've created around my illness. I've learned ways to keep a songwriter's dream alive despite having a body with a mind of its own. Despite depletion, weakness, fear, anxiety, drugs, risks, therapies, I've always had love and gratitude and humor. I've always had music and art. They are my lifelines. The creativity I've turned to again and again as a healing path has brought joy, fulfillment, and deep connections with others. I can't stop creating!

I know that not everyone can or wants to do what I'm doing. I'm simply here to share my journey and my story and show you, if you are afflicted by illness—or by anything life throws at you, for that matter—that you don't have to be a victim, that you can still have dreams and keep them alive, that art and music and other creative pursuits are beautiful paths to wellness in the truest sense of the word, and that connection with others is an important healing strategy.

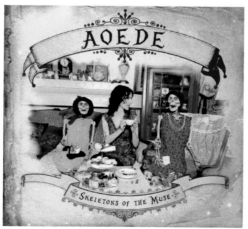

Skeletons of the Muse CD cover Apr 2012
Credit KG Photography and Oasis DesignWorks

My 2012 album, *Skeletons of the Muse*, is about coming to terms with the ghosts of my past, with my roller-coaster present, and with my uncertain future. The album cover features Aoede having tea with her skeletons, as if maybe I'm finally making friends with all they represent: my dark side, my twisting spiral staircase of a journey into chronic illness, and the vulnerability of sharing my weaknesses. My story is one of persevering through disease and disability by way of the creative process. But it's also about becoming a light in the darkness, offering support, compassion, inspiration, connection, and encouragement to those who need it most.

I didn't know that part of my journey would be sharing my story with you. But my hope is that you'll see yourself in aspects of my story, and that it will offer you the encouragement you need. Perhaps life has thrown you some curveballs, and you just want to know you're not alone as you wrestle with your feelings, thoughts, and fears. Perhaps my story will inspire you to reframe your situation, do what's in your soul, and thrive through the creative process, even if you're battling a chronic disease like mine or some other illness, or have lost your inspiration along the way. I almost did. But I've learned that while my body might be waging war against itself, my spirit cannot be crushed. Though I believe some things, such as what life throws us, are not in our control, I also believe many things are possible with the right attitude, support, creativity, and a lot of hard work and determination.

I've lived with a chronic disability for more than ten years now. Progress has been incremental, and sometimes I take one step forward only to take two steps back. Besides my rheumatologist, I've seen dermatologists, neurologists, endocrinologists, gastroenterologists, oncologists, general practitioners, gynecologists, head and neck docs, allergists, pulmonologists, physical therapists, infectious-disease docs, and ophthalmologists, as well as internists, naturopathic, alternative medicine and urgent-care docs—all to "manage" the beast I live with every day. It has been a tough road. But without it, I might never have discovered my true self and purpose and started dreaming so big in the first place. I believe that everything happens to bring each of us to the next leg of our journeys.

You see, I started as a singer-songwriter, but through all of this, I became a muse and a light in the darkness. Because of my experience, I can share, connect, and inspire. Hopefully my words, lyrics, and personal triumphs will help you find renewed strength and motivation in those moments when you don't feel like getting out of bed.

If you've lost your inspiration because of a significant change in health status, know that you can still pursue your dreams. You can live with hope, passion, and joy, even if the shape and substance of your dreams have changed. While this book chronicles my personal journey, my hope is to inspire you to consider how to view your situation from the perspective I have gained.

Being Aoede the Muse has turned out to be a gift in disguise, not just a coping mechanism propelling me through the darkness of chronic illness.

I offer this gift to you, with love.

Chapter 1

Struggling With a Body in Revolt

"Everyone has a whole other life that no one knows about."

—Pretty Little Liars

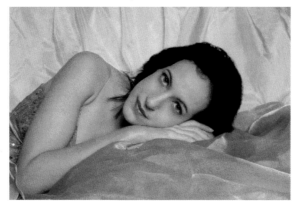

Aoede Dec 2010—Credit William Boice Photography

I'm just a kid filled with curiosity and wonder, and I still believe in fairy tales and dreams and magic. If you had asked for my bio some years ago, I would have immediately answered, "I'm Aoede, an award-winning, quirky folk-pop singer-songwriter, recording and performing artist, playwright, author, and muse." I also would have pointed you to my accolades: "Aoede has been honored with more than forty awards for songwriting, audiobooks, and stage plays since 2012." That's how I want you to see me: Aoede, the Muse of Song.

After all, isn't that what you really want to read about: the achievements; the success stories; the happy, inspirational, positive moments; the milestones; the CD releases; the performances? Don't you want to click "Like" on Facebook when I post the photo of the pretty dress I wore at the Grammy Awards? Congratulate me on my two Indie Music Channel Awards statues? Comment on my new photo-shoot pictures, or on the latest fascinator I'm wearing in my hair?

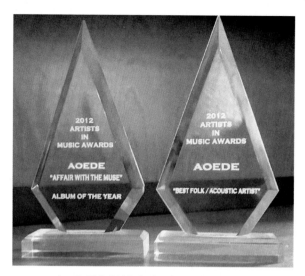

Aoede Feb 2012 Artists in Music Awards

That's what I really wanted to show you … until now. Don't get me wrong. I'm so filled with gratitude that I can experience and learn from each of these moments, and I'm crazy thrilled about every success. I live for connecting, engaging, and having family, friends, and fans share in my journey as Aoede the Muse. In my monthly online newsletters to my fans, I stick to sharing good, positive, light, bright, happy! Lots of exclamation points!!! Smiles ☺ Hearts! ◉ PLAY! Aoede the Muse is my identity. It's who I am today. It's in my childlike, quirky music. It colors my musicals and all of my art forms.

But that's not the whole story. You know that by now.

I'm really good at glossing over the day-to-day reality of living with a chronic illness. When connecting with friends and new fans, I haven't been inclined to share the price of going to award shows, workshops, and conferences; the toll of traveling to and from Los Angeles to record my music; the days of recuperation after back-to-back events; the roller coaster of endless drug cocktails and their nasty side effects; or the relentless routine of physical therapy. I haven't wanted to talk about the 156 doctors' appointments I've been to so far, the weekly pool rehab sessions, the walker and the cane I use when my legs won't hold me, the infections, the constant fatigue, and the need for rest, which is never restorative.

Before now, I wouldn't have dared divulge that while I shot day one of a music video in January 2011, I had to sit in my wheelchair between takes, and it took all my strength to walk across the room in my wobbly black platform shoes. I wouldn't have shared that driving to Los Angeles in May and July 2010 to record one of my albums, *Affair with the Muse*, was one of the few times I left my home that whole year. For sure, I wouldn't have wanted you to know I was in the hospital for more than three weeks that year. I wouldn't have told you that I have dermatomyositis (DM).

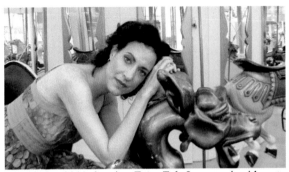

Aoede Jan 2011 shooting *Fairy Tale Love* music video at
Yerba Buena Gardens Carousel in San Francisco—Credit Eva Beck

Don't worry if you can't say it or spell it. It took me months to do so, and years to admit it. *It's my private business*, I used to think. But in July 2009, I had to take a leave of absence from my day job as an environmental scientist because of my worsening health. On top of working full time and putting energy into music and gigs, I was fighting fatigue, weakness, and infections. I was dealing with what life was handing me the best I could, pushing myself day after day, taking Western medications, and experimenting with alternative therapies, but each day I felt more and more depleted.

In my October 2010 newsletter, I alluded to health problems, commenting that I was learning to adjust to a new norm, but I was never specific about my private challenges. I didn't share the fact that I live as a disabled artist with a chronic illness. That is what I didn't tell you … until now.

The title song of my quirky folk-pop album *Skeletons of the Muse* begins with these lyrics: "Just decided that today I'll tell you what I don't want you to know. That's what I'll do."[1] Truth is, I wasn't really ready to be quite so vulnerable and to divulge my secrets when that album was released in 2012. I didn't get that it wasn't just about making the music and giving that music to you. It was and is about giving *me* to you, even the parts I want to keep buried deep inside. All the skeletons I haven't wanted you to see … until now.

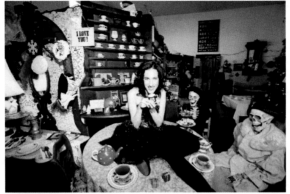

Aoede Jan 2012 *Skeletons of the Muse* photo shoot in San Francisco
Credit KG Photography and Lovejoy's Tea Room

When I was first diagnosed with DM in April 2008, lots of "life" stuff was happening, personally and professionally. There was my job as a scientist; a huge high-profile workshop I was helping plan that spring; my other full-time job as singer-songwriter, performer, and recording artist; my upcoming wedding and reception (I was marrying David, my bass player); and a tour to promote my newest CD, *Push and Pull*. It wasn't unusual for me to have so many balls in the air, but it kept me in go-go-go mode until I finally ran out of juice.

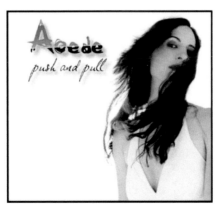

Push and Pull CD cover 2008
Credit Liz Caruana Photography and Oasis DesignWorks

Ironically, it was before all these events, just before the big workshop and only a few weeks before the wedding, that I noticed I had a rash on both hands, along with red nail beds and knuckles, and cuticles that were painful to the touch. I recall the pain of doing simple things like washing dishes or pulling items out of my backpack. My hands always felt hot, and at times incredibly itchy, but it was manageable. Mostly I was self-conscious, wore gloves, and hid my hands a lot.

I went to the dermatologist thinking he would prescribe a cortizone cream for what was probably contact dermatitis or something else that could easily be cured. But when he saw me, he immediately diagnosed me with DM because of the telltale rash on my hands. Some people go years without getting accurately diagnosed, especially later in the course of their disease when they present with symptoms like muscle pain or weakness that mimic other illnesses.

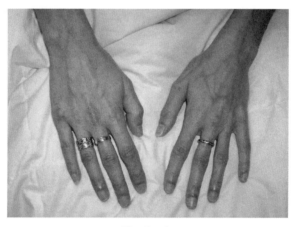

Hand rash

During what I thought would be a fairly routine doctor's appointment, I was plunged into a world that was completely foreign, and I didn't want to know about. I learned that dermatomyositis is an inflammatory condition (itis) of the skin (derma) and muscles (myo). It's a connective-tissue disease in which the immune system attacks and destroys healthy skin and muscles instead of just fighting infection or viruses the way it's supposed to. Underlying causes for DM are unknown, but it may result from a viral infection or an autoimmune reaction.

The incidence of DM in the United States is estimated at around 9.63 cases per million people.[2] DM is twice as common in women than in men.

The main symptoms include skin rash and symmetrical, proximal muscle weakness (which basically means the muscles closest to and within the trunk of the body get progressively weaker), with the neck, hips, shoulders, and legs most affected. Since there is no cure for DM, one of the key medical treatments is immunosuppression, which inhibits the inflammatory attack on the skin, muscles, and other body systems.

Between April and June 2008, after I was diagnosed, I had a series of blood tests and a skin biopsy, started prednisone to keep my immune system from attacking my skin, continued to work, got married, and prepared for my Aoede artist tour. I tried to ignore what my body was telling me, yet I was faced with constant reminders that something was wrong. I started hiding my red knuckles and nail beds and covering my chest and arms—and eventually my legs and feet—so the rash wouldn't peek through. I was afraid the rash would never go away.

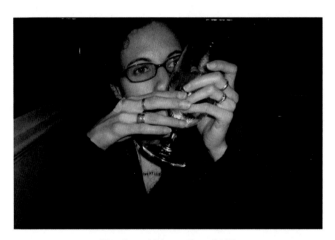

Hands and biopsy June 2008

Each time I went through screening tests—CT scans, mammograms, ultrasounds—I was reminded that I could have cancer or other medical issues associated with DM. There are so many things to be afraid of when doctors keep reminding you of everything there might be to fear!

In late June, David and I went on tour as Aoede, driving through California and up through Oregon and Washington. It was a hot summer in the Pacific Northwest, and I was in the sun more often. That's when I noticed the rash was spreading to other parts of my body, and I was becoming more tired. Apparently, I was learning the hard way: heat and sun can exacerbate symptoms of DM. I talked to my cousin Gary, a naturopathic doctor in Oregon, who convinced me to modify my diet. Gluten, for example, can cause inflammation and make skin problems worse. So come July, when I returned home, I stopped eating many foods that have been linked to inflammation.

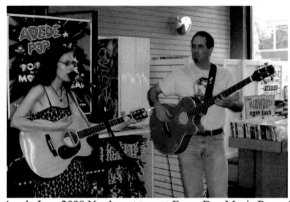

Aoede June 2008 Northwest tour at Every Day Music Record Store
Bellingham, WA with David Sands

Nevertheless, come October 2008, I noticed I was having difficulty lifting my arms in the shower, brushing my hair, putting on my backpack, climbing stairs, and even getting up from the couch. My upper-body weakness was becoming more severe. At first I thought it was psychosomatic—I knew that some people with DM had muscle weakness, so maybe I was imagining it. But after a few months of increased weakness and fatigue, I had more blood work, an EMG (electromyography), and an MRI, all of which confirmed that my abnormal muscle activity and inflammation were consistent with a DM diagnosis.

My rheumatologist strongly recommended that I start an immunosuppressive drug called methotrexate, since my skin and muscle inflammation didn't seem to be responding to the meds prescribed thus far. I was getting weaker and weaker, so I sought out anything that might make me feel better, including alternative therapies. But while having a massage, for instance, I couldn't even keep my arms on the table. Everything was so tender to the touch that the therapist had to be extra gentle. What would normally relax me wiped me out!

As a scientist, I'm pretty analytical and have an obsessive desire to learn everything I can about areas that interest me. DM was no exception. I hit the

Internet and then the library to learn what I could about the latest studies on DM (which were few, especially longitudinal—over time—studies) and the types of treatments available. I was resistant to the idea of what I considered toxic drugs. In the course of my research, as well as time spent in chat rooms and at local support-group meetings, I discovered that many people need to take immunosuppressive drugs for many years, if not for life, to keep DM under control. At that point, I wasn't ready to ingest noxious drugs long term, so I soldiered ahead. I could feel the pain and weakness, but I fought tooth and nail to keep working, performing, and pursuing my dreams, my body be damned.

But my skin rash persisted, and as my muscles got progressively weaker, I lost weight and muscle mass. I was not only seeing my rheumatologist more, but I was also getting monthly blood work, being monitored for cancer, and doing physical therapy. I got a second opinion from a dermatologist who specialized in DM, and he convinced me that left on its own, and considering how active my DM was, this disease could leave me bedridden, or worse, from muscle wasting and uncontrolled inflammation. I finally agreed to start immunosuppressive treatment: the dreaded methotrexate.

I continued working after starting the drug, which I took once a week, but I worked more and more from home. I noticed that commuting by public transit was getting really difficult, and I was incredibly fatigued all the time, especially on the days I took the drug. I never felt rested no matter how much sleep I got. My hair was falling out too.

Despite my health issues, some exciting developments were taking place on the music front: my song "I Lost, You Win" was featured on American Airlines; Aoede was WomensRadio's Top Artist of 2008; and my album *Push and Pull* was being distributed in stores, added to radio-station playlists nationwide, and getting great reviews. Our band played ten shows from January to March 2009. We went to Nashville for an industry showcase in April. We shot the remainder of the music video *I Lost, You Win* in one day in July. And we played or scheduled twenty-one shows from May to December. Those were a *lot* of gigs, even for a healthy person, and all of it required energy I simply didn't have.

My body finally revolted. I was forced to quit my full-time job in July 2009 and had to cancel gigs. I just couldn't get through the days anymore without extreme depletion and brain fog. And then there was the fun of multiple infections because my immune system was so suppressed. It was getting harder and harder for me to be in public. Nevertheless, in spite of fatigue, weakness, biopsies, endless blood work, infections, and fifty-three doctor's appointments from April 2008 through December 2009, I was determined to focus my limited energy on my music. I pondered who I was as an artist and realized that it wasn't just about the songs; it was about making connections with my friends, touching my fans, and not being afraid to be vulnerable or reveal myself to them, at least through my music.

At my last show in December 2009, I began by standing and singing; then midway through the concert, I had to sit, ultimately cutting my set list because I just didn't have any more energy. It was then I had to admit I wasn't getting better. I couldn't perform without it totally wiping me out. I was on a downward spiral and was wrestling more and more with questions like these: *What will become of my dreams if I can no longer perform? How can I realize my dreams when my body keeps resisting, protesting, and begging me to slow down and stop?*

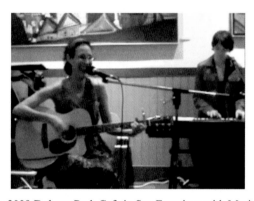

Aoede Dec 2009 Dolores Park Cafe in San Francisco with Marianna Ferris

Methotrexate kept me on a roller coaster—some mild improvement in the weakness, I thought; a lot of side effects; and a lot more infections. From August through December, I had to cancel or turn down a growing number of gigs.

Nevertheless, I still wasn't listening to my body. I wanted to do all the things I had previously been able to do when I was healthy. My idea of success was to go full steam ahead, fire on all cylinders all the time, and achieve whatever I could dream up. My imagination was soaring. My body was rebelling.

Looking back, I have no idea how I managed to juggle my art, let alone life, with the war my body was waging. Honestly, I think I saw only what I wanted to see. I didn't want to focus entirely on my body; I wanted to have exciting, inspiring reasons to get up each morning. There was just no way I would let DM get the best of me! I lived by former NFL player Chad Williams's motto: "Life's only limitations are those you set upon yourself, for as long as you strive hard enough, anything is achievable." If I could dream *anything* and work hard to make it happen, then I could dream away this disease. I could heal myself if only I dreamed big enough and believed hard enough.

I had always worked hard. And I dreamed big. When I envisioned something that might be, I asked how I could make it so. Surely I could do the same thing with this illness. I had to. I was too afraid to see what might become of me if the music was indeed changing.

Chapter 2
Acknowledging Limitations

"I try not to worry about the future ...
so I take each day just one anxiety attack at a time."

—Tom Wilson, *Ziggyisms*

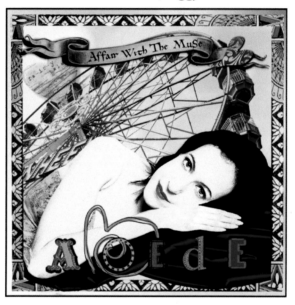

Affair with the Muse 2011 CD cover

B etween January and June 2010, I was doing all I could to keep up my strength despite my increasing muscle weakness, skin rash, fatigue, and a barrage of immunosuppressive treatments that totally wiped me out for days at a time. Each day I would nap, sometimes multiple times. I did some light weight-bearing therapy to strengthen my arms and aqua therapy once a week. Nearly every day I walked around the block in my neighborhood, sometimes making a game out of spotting something new each time—a row of flowers, a sculpture, a cool awning. Rather than resist taking my medicines, I tried to accept them as something that would help me. I kept to a strict gluten-free, sugar-free, dairy-free diet. I was willing to do anything to boost my energy and stamina and get my health back. But it seemed like a moving target.

Food didn't seem to want to go down as easily as it used to. I had little appetite and kept losing weight. I also had a lot of questions:

Why was I having trouble swallowing?

Why was I so brain fogged and sleeping so much?

Were these symptoms of the disease or side effects of the medicine?

I don't think anybody could have predicted back then what would happen next.

If I had to sum up what was floating around in my head space from June through August 2010, three words would have been my mantra: *Just ... keep ... going. Keep doing everything I can to not think about what was happening. Just ... keep ... going ... until*—well, I didn't know until what. At the time, those words—Just ... keep ... going—were stuck on repeat like a broken record.

I was constantly in 'go' mode, even organizing material and collaborators to put together an artistic-innovation grant for 2011. My project, *Alice in Waterland*, used story, music, and film to connect Bay Area teens with their watersheds. As an environmental scientist, I had put my heart and soul into California coastal water-quality protection, working for two state agencies for nearly ten years. When I left work in 2009, I had combined my two passions—music and water—into a rock-pop-style coastal anthem directed at kids titled "Blue Gold." It was intended to celebrate our precious liquid resources and raise awareness of the impact of plastics and marine debris. It was my way of continuing to effect change and stay in the game even though I was clearly unable to work.

A music-strategy guru gave me the idea to create a small book of illustrated lyrics to accompany the new single. There was so much more to tell kids about the ocean, water, pollution, plastics, and toxins. I decided I wanted to write not only more water-themed pop music but also a children's or teens' water-themed book covering different water topics.

I was buoyed by the idea of submitting a grant for a water project that wouldn't materialize until far in the future. Surely by 2011, I would have kicked DM to the curb and could, in the meantime, focus on a creative and worthwhile project. Another part of me shuddered at the thought of being awarded a grant. How would I be able to implement it given the hand I was dealt? I couldn't work; I couldn't drive; I couldn't even leave the house most days for lack of stamina. I was still losing weight and having trouble swallowing. When pieces of food did go down, I didn't digest them well. Even my breathing was affected.

At the same time, my muse was flowing and took the form of a few new pop songs that would eventually be part of my next album, *Affair with the Muse*. Earlier in March of 2010, I connected with a producer in Los Angeles named Scrote, who expressed interest in working with me and planted the seeds for me to record in the summer. But as summer approached, I kept asking myself how I would get through such energy-intense recording days.

The recording experience turned out to be incredibly positive because I was fulfilling a dream. But it was also terribly exhausting. I mustered all the strength I had to give it my best, but my husband David had to pick me up from the chair after just two hours of work because I was so weak. By the end of the second day, I couldn't complete the vocals on one song and had to record them later at a different studio closer to home.

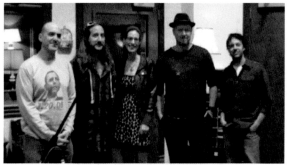

Aoede recording May 2010 Eldorado Studio Burbank, CA
With David Piltch, Dave Palmer, Scrote, Blair Sinta

In spite of the toll DM was taking on my body, I was inspired to write a few new songs. One of these songs, "What You Got," became my personal anthem. When life is hurling lemons at you, when you're so tired you can't get out of bed, whatever life throws at you, you've got to pick yourself up and do what you can with what you've got! I wrote this song to instill hope in myself and perhaps to encourage others who were encountering unforeseen challenges. Little did I know that my greatest challenge was just ahead.

At the end of August and again in early September, I had appointments with a GI specialist to evaluate my digestive issues, pain, and continued weight loss. They scheduled an endoscopy for mid-September.

By September 4, I couldn't swallow very well, even without food. I felt extra lethargic and decided a walk around the block would revive me.

When I returned home, my mouth felt particularly dry, and I reached for a glass of water. For several seconds I was unable to swallow. There was pain and clicking in my throat, and I couldn't make saliva. My words were slurred and took a lot of effort. I spoke unnaturally, very mechanically, like a robot, and wasn't able to connect my words. I couldn't think straight. I tried to stand, but I couldn't lift my body. I actually checked my legs to make sure I could still feel them. My heart was racing.

David and I decided the ER was probably the right place to go. When I woke up on that Friday morning, September 4, 2010, in my regular bed, I didn't know I wouldn't be sleeping in it that evening, let alone see our house again for more than three weeks!

I remember only a few details of that night, such as having an IV, blood tests, and a CT scan; not being allowed to drink and feeling incredibly thirsty; and finally being admitted the next morning after many hours of waiting. The doctors were scrambling to figure out what was happening.

I learned quickly that hospitals are not places of rest. Nurses, doctors, a dietician, a social worker, and other staff came and went at all hours of the day and night, introducing themselves and telling me who would be attending to me. I was so out of it and tired but don't remember sleeping much because someone was constantly there to take my blood pressure, temperature, and blood; stick monitors on my body; administer medicine; ask me questions; and of course, give me a bedpan, since I couldn't get up. I felt so dependent and embarrassed.

My rheumatologist came in to consult with me on a plan. I agreed to high-dose prednisone for at least three days. We would do neurological tests, work on the swallowing, and get that endoscopy the gastroenterologist had recommended. It seemed as if I was constantly being shuttled back and forth between tests and procedures, catching sleep whenever I could.

After a few days on the prednisone, I still wasn't able to stand and had no strength in my upper and lower body. I was moved to the ICU and given another immunosuppressive biological drug for five days while being closely monitored. I didn't notice any difference in strength after the treatment. I wore leg-compression stockings and was given daily heparin shots to prevent blood clots from inactivity. Various therapists came to my room and worked with me on sitting up and moving to the edge of the bed, with assistance from transfer belts to keep me from falling over. Everything took so much energy!

And I had such a short attention span. I don't recall being online or reading anything for weeks.

My mom was with me at the hospital day in and day out for twenty-four days. Sometimes when you're in a strange place with strangers around you, having your mom with you is the best therapy there is. David would visit each night after work so Mom could go home and get some sleep. During the first few days, Mom and David traded shifts overnight, because being on all that heavy medicine left me jittery and more anxious than usual. My sister-in-law, Helen, and David's parents also visited frequently, as did friends.

It seemed that someone was always there with me, surrounding me with love despite my inability to hold conversations. I couldn't do much but surrender—allow the doctors and nurses to treat me; allow young male nurses to bathe me in bed or help me to the commode; allow myself to be poked and prodded; stop trying to control much of anything. It was as if it wasn't me going through all the motions. It felt surreal, and I was barely present.

Though doctors couldn't confirm that DM had caused all my symptoms, eventually, my caseworker recommended intensive rehabilitation involving several hours a day of physical, occupational, and speech therapy. At first I just wanted to go home; the idea of spending more time in the hospital held no appeal, especially since the rehab hospital was nearly two hours from where we lived. But the fact was, I was barely able to stand for more than thirty seconds at a time.

Independence is such an integral part of who I am. Prior to DM, if I needed food, I could walk or drive somewhere to eat or pick up groceries. If I needed to go to a doctor's appointment, I could take myself. If friends asked David and me to come over, we could do that. If we wanted to go away for a few days or to a show or to see some exhibit in San Francisco, it was no problem. But now I was dependent on David and my mom for all my basic needs. Talk about loss of dignity and identity!

When I began to face the reality of where I was in terms of my dependence and what it would be like at home without any accommodations to get around the house, cook, bathe, or even go to the bathroom, I decided it would be too much of a burden for Mom and David. I opted to go to rehab.

I was transported to the rehab hospital by ambulance and gurney on September 16, 2010, my parents' anniversary date. I hoped it was the first and last time I'd have to travel by ambulance! Once I arrived at the new hospital, Mom and David helped unpack familiar things that made my room feel homier. They filled my drawers with snacks Mom brought to give me a break from orange, green, and white food, since I was on a soft, extra-restricted diet. They also showered me with other little gifts, such as pretty pajamas to wear instead of the hospital gown that barely covered my backside. They placed everything within reach, since I was too weak to get up.

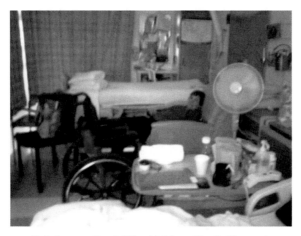

Rehab room Sep 2010 with Mom (Jan Sniderman)

I didn't require medical monitoring around the clock like I did at the other hospital, but everything was measured: what and how much I ate, and what came out! I also got my first shower in thirteen days. I was wheeled into the bathroom on a big chair that sat right under the stream of water. Even with the nurses helping me, I felt so wiped out afterward.

I was issued my very own wheelchair (oh, joy) and had to wear a yellow FALL RISK bracelet at all times. Since I couldn't stand without wobbling, I had to transfer from the bed to the chair with the assistance of a nurse. I wondered how long it would be before I could go to the bathroom by myself.

When I first got to the new hospital, I thought rehabilitation would happen quickly. I thought I'd be there for only a weekend or two and then walk out the door and go back to my old life. I was just waiting for the drugs to kick in. But the therapy was grueling. All I remember thinking was *How on earth am I going to be able to stay awake through all of this?* I had slept most of the day at the other hospital; now I was expected to do various therapies for thirty to forty-five minutes at a time!

As I anticipated, I didn't make it through the first day of therapy. I did try to do what was asked in physical therapy, but I was exhausted by the time

I hit speech therapy and couldn't even sit through the swallowing session, where I was supposed to try eating. I felt like a battery that had only a small charge left.

Over the next weeks, everything was about energy conservation. If I had a shower in the morning, I needed to rest until therapy. When I had one therapy session, I needed to rest until the next one. If I had visitors … You guessed it. I didn't want to imagine the road ahead: weeks or months of therapy and rehabilitation. I had so much work to do just to get to a new baseline that involved wheelchairs, ramps, walkers, canes, a commode, and shower seats.

Occupational-therapy staff would come to my room and help me with activities of daily living, like helping me figure out how to get my socks on and whether to brush my teeth or wash my face when I was too tired to do both. In physical therapy, therapists would show me stretches and help pull and push my legs and arms when they didn't seem to want to move on their own. I would get so exhausted and have to rest back in my room. Then another occupational-therapy session followed, where I was given games to play to improve my hand grip and strength. In speech therapy, I focused on food and swallowing issues. How strange it felt to spend some sessions just trying different textures! We also focused on concentration, since I couldn't focus on anything for long. I was given memory-and brain-booster computer games to help.

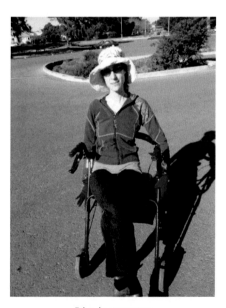

Lisa in recovery

The last physical-therapy session of the day was the hardest for me. They called it *gait therapy*. I was supposed to walk as many steps as I could with the support of a walker. I'm pretty obedient, and also pretty determined, and I would do as they asked. However, I quickly realized that it was too much. I would be so exhausted that I would collapse and then have no energy to eat or do much else for several hours. So the staff decided to schedule my gait work earlier in the day and ask a little less of me.

As the days went by, I was able to stand with assistance and take a few more steps with the walker, but I tired so quickly! One day I finally had a breakthrough. I told my occupational therapist that I was a singer-songwriter, and I wanted to be able to play my guitar and sing again. He asked David to bring my Martin acoustic guitar to the hospital, which he did, but this special therapist also brought his kid's guitar, maybe two-thirds the size of a standard guitar, for me to play. Even that small guitar was hard for me to hold, and I could barely play or even sing because my entire core and even my vocal cords were so weak. But just having that guitar in my hands and whispering the familiar lyrics to "What You Got" renewed something in me. For the first time since entering the hospital, I thought, *I'm going to be okay. I will get through this. And this is what I've got to give right now.*

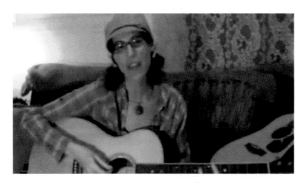

Lisa Jul 2011 in recovery

When I finally returned home from the rehab hospital in late September 2010, my bed, my couch, and I became the best of friends. For the first few months, I was confined to a wheelchair even to get around my house. I couldn't walk more than a few steps without weakness and exhaustion. David, my sister, or my mom, depending who was around, made me daily protein shakes because I had lost so much weight and muscle mass in the hospital and still had swallowing issues. A nurse's aide came to bathe me several times each week, and physical and occupational therapists worked with me at home from October through December on simple activities like holding my neck and head up for more than thirty seconds at a time, doing exercises in my chair, or increasing my hand and core strength. Eventually, with a lot of effort, I gained strength, started to stand, and then began walking with a walker and then a cane. Finally, I was able to hold my guitar again.

For the next six months, from October 2010 to April 2011, I was on a combination of different drugs, therapies, and treatments, all to manage my illness and give me the best quality of life possible. The problem was that the drugs, on top of my autoimmune disease, created additional side effects and new health problems that set me back in my recovery. I was constantly on edge, watching for any new ailment that crept up, so I could monitor it before it triggered another DM flare-up, which was my worst fear.

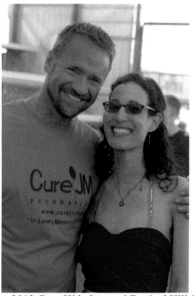

Aoede Aug 2012 Cure Kids Jam and Festival Hillsboro, OR
with Organizer Damon Smedley

The other issue, which continued for years after my hospital stay, was that I didn't want to listen to my body and tended to do too much, which would also result in setbacks. To illustrate, I plunged myself into a whirlwind of nonstop music-related activities in 2012. I ignored my body's increasing weakness and continually fought taking my daily nap. In January of that year, I was prepping for the release of another album and walking unassisted at home. In February, I spoke on a conference panel as a do-it-yourself indie artist, accepted two music awards in Los Angeles, and then returned home to have an infusion of a new drug called Rituxan. In April, I released a video and new album and returned to Los Angeles for more music awards. In June, I held a CD-and-music-video-release party, where I sang in public for the first time in nearly a year. In July, I sang the national anthem at a baseball game. In August, David and I traveled to talk and perform at a festival for an organization called Cure JM Foundation, which focuses on finding a cure for kids with juvenile myositis (JM) and improving the lives of families affected by the disease. In September, I released my first musical-story audiobook CD and performed in Los Angeles for an LA music-awards voting party. In November, David and I attended a music-industry conference and then another awards show in Los Angeles.

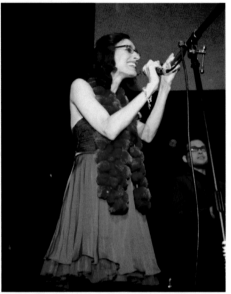

Aoede Feb 2012 accepting Artists in Music Awards in Los Angeles, CA
Credit Mickey Yeh

In December 2012, I was supposed to return to Los Angeles to accept nominations for the Artists in Music Awards and was determined to be there. No surprise, I piled on too many back-to-back activities (three trips over three consecutive weekends) and ended up getting sick. So instead of receiving the nominations in person, my PR folks had to accept them on my behalf. Even after that, I kept ignoring what my body was telling me: SLOW DOWN!

It wasn't long before I overdid it and got sick again … and again and again. I kept hoping I was getting better and would have more stamina for the things I wanted to do, but I had no way of knowing what was too much until my body told me by getting sick and giving me no choice but to stop doing nearly everything. I kept pushing and going, probably to convince myself that even though I had DM, DM wouldn't have me!

In time, however, I had to come to terms with the fact that I wasn't in control of my body anymore; it marched to its own drumbeat now. I had to surrender my denial and resistance and start making peace with my limitations. It was like bursting the proverbial bubble—or finding out there's no Santa Claus. It meant facing that I wasn't invincible. I couldn't just do whatever I set my mind to.

Accepting that I had limitations was even harder than accepting I had DM. But I had to learn to embrace the drill: go to an event. Nap. Go to another event. Rest some more. Skip some things because even though my mind wanted to do everything, my body said no. This was my new normal—always having to choose one thing over another, not both. The music had indeed changed, and I had to find a new dance.

Chapter 3
Redefining Success

"Success is not a place at which one arrives, but rather the spirit with which one undertakes and continues the journey."

—Alex Noble

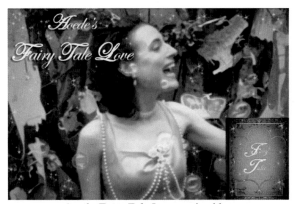

Aoede *Fairy Tale Love* music video
Credit Eva Beck

How I define and measure success has been a moving target during different stages of my life. When I was working full time as an environmental scientist, I measured success in terms of pay-scale advancement or increasing job responsibilities or even my ability to pay my own rent and bills and live independently after separating from my first husband and before David and I moved in together. When I was forced to quit working in 2009 because of increasing debilitation from DM, I struggled with both my identity and my view of success. I heard two conflicting messages in my head. From my mom: "You can be and do anything!" and from my dad: "As long as you get a trade!"

Both of my parents expected me to go to college and groomed me for it. I was eager to go. I've always loved learning, and I enjoyed the academic challenges of high school despite the awkwardness of being a teenager and wearing different hats for four years to figure out who I was becoming while trying my best to fit in. After taking mostly advanced prep classes and earning excellent grades in high school, I was accepted as a freshman at the University of California. My parents supported me through my undergraduate degree at UC Santa Barbara and UC Santa Cruz, with Dad's "Get a trade" message fueling my drive and passion to get my BA and later my master's in environmental studies. My concentration was water-quality protection and watershed management. I also minored in sociology because I found the sociology of natural resources fascinating. I was interested in the many ways people relate to a public resource like water, so when I later got a job creating and implementing water-quality policy for the State of California, it was a good fit for my experience and interests and kept my analytical mind challenged.

When I realized I could no longer work because of DM, I had an identity crisis. I didn't know how I would effect change or be a contributing member of society when I was sick at home and drawing disability income. Even though music was my business, I saw wearing my singer-songwriter hat or doing my art as a hobby, something that brought me pleasure and joy on the side, while my "real" job was working as an environmental scientist. Sometimes I still think that if I got better and could work again, I would have to return to that job and the fast-paced nine-to-five, go-go-go city life. I've struggled with owning that I'm an artist, seeing my art as a beautiful contribution all by itself and letting that be good enough—for me, for society, and I guess for my parents.

I've had a lot to learn about myself—mostly, what success is to me and how I measure it. All of us have different journeys and different stars that guide us. I had to learn that I didn't need to compare myself with anyone. I had my own path and dreams, and it was my job to find new ways to make them come true, in spite of the fact I qualified for Social Security Disability at the age of thirty-seven.

Isn't it interesting how we tend to focus on what we fail to accomplish rather than on all we actually achieve? When I look back at 2010 and 2011, post-hospital, I can't believe how much I accomplished despite my limitations. From the time I arrived home from my twenty-four-day hospital stay, I was trying to figure out how to get the music I had recorded in 2010 out into the world—all while physical and occupational therapists were coming to the house multiple times a week, while family and friends shuttled me back and forth each month to the hospital for IV immunoglobulin (IVIG) infusions (which had been shown to be effective for controlling some DM cases), and while I was learning a new norm that required the assistance of medical equipment. When six new music tracks were completed prehospital, I had checked in with my distribution company to see how to release them. Next thing I knew, by December that year, I found myself retaining and working with a PR firm on a new bio and press release, developing a new website, setting up a photo shoot and getting new photos, and taking up ukulele and recording a seventh song that would be included on the new EP (extended-play album).

In late January 2011, I shot a music video for "Fairy Tale Love," the first track from my new album, to get the live action shots. The shoot took place at three locations over three days: inside a mechanical museum, on a carousel, and outside our house in our gardens. At the museum I was very weak and was still using my wheelchair for transport; yet somehow I managed, with the help of my videographer, Eva, to sing along with the sound track, muster my strength to walk in platform shoes, and hold myself upright, using the fortune-telling machines for balance long enough for her to capture each of the necessary shots. Between shots I had to rest in my wheelchair and regain my strength. We were at the museum for what seemed like hours!

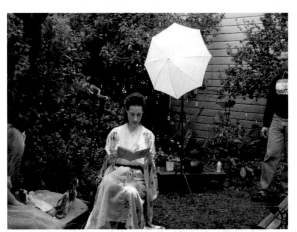

Making of *Fairy Tale Love*, Jan 2011 San Francisco
with Elena O'Kane and David Sands

At the carousel I had very little stamina, but I rode the painted horses and dragons up and down and sang my song aloud while we went around and around to get the shots. My weakened body hadn't had that many thrills in years!

The shoot at home required a team consisting of Eva, David and me, David's sister, Helen (costumer extraordinaire), a hair-and-makeup artist, and friends. It was a low budget production, but very involved, with a lot of prep work for sets, costumes, hair and makeup, lighting, and music syncing. Though I was exhausted at every turn, my head and heart were happy to be creating. My vision for the video was that an animated fairy-tale book would fall from the sky and flip open, inviting viewers to come play along, as if they were transported into a magical fairy-tale world. The video would also flip back and forth between live action and animation.

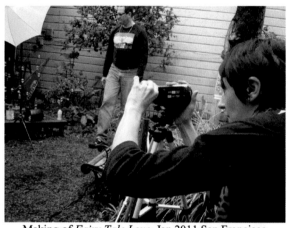

Making of *Fairy Tale Love*, Jan 2011 San Francisco
with Eva Beck and David Sands

I had some setbacks and had to find new collaborators midway through production because of creative differences and logistical challenges. It took more than a year to manifest, but "Fairy Tale Love" planted the seeds for me to later create my first musical-story audiobook for tweens, *Is Love a Fairy Tale?* Watching the completed music video, you would never know I had been in the hospital for nearly a month only four months before.

In February 2011, while still getting monthly IVIG infusions, I launched my new website and started my first blog. I also began engaging with new fans on Twitter, Facebook, and other social networks, and I released my first music video *I Lost, You Win*. I released my album *Affair with the Muse* digitally in March 2011, and throughout 2011, continued to write and record more songs for a new album and engage fans through social networking, worked on completing my music video, gave radio interviews, won a music contest, was nominated for indie music awards, successfully funded a Kickstarter for my next album in December, and licensed songs. Except for parts of the music-video shoot, I did all of this from home—mostly from bed!

Between 2012 and 2018, I received more than fifty awards for my songwriting, stage plays, audiobooks, and music videos. To be bestowed with honors and recognition is beyond amazing to me. It reflected the caliber of the music I was creating and releasing and my hard work in the face of all my DM limitations. It also gave me hope, confidence, and inspiration to keep pursuing my dreams and affirmed that I was on the right path—that my music was having an impact.

However, I've had to learn not to base my worth on whether or not I win or achieve. Awards do not equal success and won't take away my illness. Awards won't satisfy my need to create and connect and effect change. I am paving my own path. This is my journey, and no one else can take it for me.

In July 2010, just before my DM flared up and sent me to the hospital, I wrote down some pretty ambitious goals in my journal, including the following:

* Write a fantasy novel for young adults.

* Write and record new Aoede pop music.

* Promote and market new singles.

* Record four new children's water-themed songs.

* Submit grant for *Alice in Waterland* project.

* Spend quality time with David.

* Keep good communication with friends and family.

I also listed some smaller goals: ways to improve my energy and stamina incrementally. I became more and more realistic about what I could and couldn't do. I decided it was enough to walk around my neighborhood every day for just fifteen minutes and do ten minutes of arm-strengthening exercises every other day. It was okay to take one-to-two-hour naps and embrace this as part of my new-normal day.

My big goals keep me dreaming, but the small ones keep me grounded. It isn't about reaching all my goals; it's about having them in the first place and realizing that by simply offering myself and my work to the world, I might connect with people and make an impact in my own unique way.

It's taken time to learn that success can be measured in so many ways besides how many records I sell, how many awards I receive, or how many music tours I have under my belt. I've learned that my art—and my life— doesn't have to fit into a nice, neat little box with a road map to the top so I'll know when I've arrived. For me, becoming willing to share the reality of my journey with others—not just the happy and light moments, but the dips and dives, the dark twists along the way, the rejections, the disappointments, the fears and doubts—is a kind of success in itself. Now, whenever I find myself dwelling on what I can no longer do, I remind myself of all I still can do and have done while living with DM. I'm always growing as an artist and a person, and this knowledge helps me remain encouraged and grateful with each passing year.

Chapter 4
Facing Your Fears

"Face your fears and doubts, and new worlds will open to you."
—Robert Kiyosaki, *Rich Dad's Cashflow Quadrant*

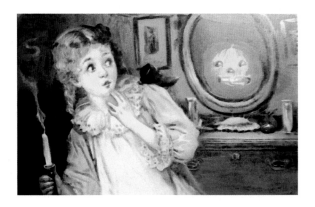

*F*ear. I often wonder how I've let such a small word have so much power over me. It's taken me years to realize that many of my feelings, thought patterns, behaviors, and motivations are actually symptoms of fear. I didn't understand that this fear has both controlled and limited the way I think and act. I couldn't confront or change what I didn't even know I was hiding behind. I'm still learning to turn off the negative messages, remind myself of my worth and value, and push and challenge myself in new ways by taking chances, feeling the fear and doing things anyway despite my disease.

I recently took a ninety-day online challenge course to help motivate me and give me some new tools and resources for writing and licensing my music. The course included inspirational mini-courses to help me break free from my fears, pursue my dreams and passions, and find my purpose. "Fearlessly Alive"[3] explored various fears, such as the fears of rejection, failure, and the unknown, and the feelings associated with them. I found myself mentally checking the symptoms of each and discovered that my greatest fears are of rejection and the unknown.

It makes so much sense. I think about my relentless pursuit of awards; my need to hold myself and others to the highest, sometimes impossible, standards; my tendency to base my self-worth on the approval of others because I care so deeply what they think of me; and my need for validation. Fear of rejection often seems to motivate me. I've had many successes and accolades, but I've had failures and disappointments too. Rejection has come in so many forms: not being awarded grants, not being chosen for productions or theater residencies, not being selected for music placement for film or television, having productions indefinitely delayed, and more. Now I can see why I'd get so disappointed or feel dejected in the past. Not achieving my goals was connected to my fear of rejection.

The online course prompted me to consider events in my life that might have set this fear in motion. I realized I've always leaned toward people pleasing, and perhaps from an early age, I learned to associate achievement, like good grades and positive performance, with love, attention, and even my worth as a person.

I believe my long hospital stay was the catalyst that brought my deepest fears to the surface. I was completely dependent, unable to perform even the most basic tasks, let alone perform music. All I could see was a shell of my former self, and I wondered whether I would ever again have the enthusiasm and physical ability to sing and play music like I used to do. (Maybe a little fear of failure was involved as well.) Perhaps as I was recovering, I threw myself into my music to prove to myself I could do it, but I also needed validation from others to motivate me to create. I needed to please others and know I was still worthy in their eyes. Maybe I donned Aoede the Muse as my public persona and wore my fascinators and pretty dresses to hide my fear that no one would like or accept the real me anymore, a disabled artist who still needed a wheelchair and a walker to get around. Going even deeper, perhaps being me wasn't good enough. Maybe I was no longer worthy of success or even fulfilling my dreams because I wasn't the same person I was before DM took my independence and introduced me to a whole new kind of vulnerability.

Besides rejection, I fear the unknown, particularly loss or change in security, support, and safety. In a worst-case scenario, being forced to work to maintain financial security could further stress my body, make my DM flare up, and land me back in the hospital, undoing years of recovery. I imagine losing my support, my gift of time, and my ability to live in my place of joy and focus on my art each day. I worry that I could change as a person— that I could lose my drive, my passions, my heart, and my spirit and have no room or interest to chase or follow my dreams if I were constantly stressed and concerned about making ends meet or getting sicker. I think of the negative impact such losses could have on my relationships with David and other family members, friends, and even fans. I can't help but wonder if I even fear success because of what it might cost me. Do I use DM as a crutch at times to avoid facing my fears? Is holding on so tightly to security and safety keeping me from even wanting to take big risks to achieve my dreams?

Perhaps the most difficult part of my journey so far has been my struggle with faith in the midst of my fear. I consider myself Jewish in terms of my identity, upbringing, and culture. Although I was brought up secular, our family celebrated Jewish rituals and holidays, and I was active in my Jewish youth group throughout high school. I even went to Jewish leadership summer camps and to Israel Summer Institute for six weeks just before my senior year. I attribute my introduction to melody and song in part to the songs and prayers the cantor would lead us in singing at temple during Friday-night services.

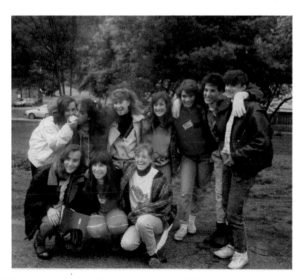

BBYO Jewish Leadership Convention 1989 San Francisco Bay Area

But in college, I wrestled with my beliefs. I remember reading some spiritual text in an essay for an environmental-ethics class and wincing every time the word *God* or *Jesus* was mentioned. I think I wrote a paper on why I was so troubled: I didn't know what I believed, and perhaps seeing something in print that claimed to be absolute truth triggered my fear that I wouldn't find what was true for me.

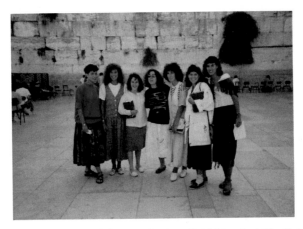

BBYO Jul 1989 Israel Summer Institute Bat Mitzvah at The Kotel

After I was diagnosed with DM, I struggled to make sense of my illness, especially without a strong faith foundation. I was facing years of unknown treatments and had a lot of fear about continuously being a guinea pig for doctors and their drugs. I was afraid of how my body might respond long term. As my illness progressed, I recognized the treatments weren't working, and I started to wrestle with life and death. I feared looking inward and confronting my darkest places. I feared death, probably because I had nothing to turn to in my faith that would allow me to come to terms with its finality. My analytical mind had no tools to study death the way I might research a new treatment. I wasn't ready to get sicker, and I wasn't ready to die. I didn't understand or accept as truth the Judeo-Christian view of death and the afterlife, but I desperately wanted to believe there was something more after death, that our bodies—our life suits—might be discarded in the cold darkness beneath the earth, but our souls would live on, and our lights would never be extinguished. More than anything, I needed to have reasons to get up each day, especially if I remained this sick.

Meditation proved to be essential in facing my fears without letting them overpower me. Because I was prone to anxiety and brain fog from all the "toxic" medications swimming around in my body, I began meditating as an exercise to calm myself. When I began receiving IVIG, it meant getting infusions one week a month for six months. I always started each infusion with a guided audio meditation and then played my recorded music or listened to instrumental music for hours through my headphones while I received treatment. When I found myself in dark, scary places, meditation enabled me to consciously stir up every negative thing I was holding on to and let it go.

During one meditation session, I finally discovered my core personal truths: "I am exactly where I need to be," and "I have everything I will ever need." These became my mantras over the next several years. They allowed me to release some of my need for control over things that were out of my control and surrender to the infusions.

Interestingly, realizing I'm not in full control hasn't led to more fear, because I hear another voice inside saying, *"Just because you fear it happening doesn't mean it's going to happen."* I still say these words to myself over and over when I'm riding in an elevator or feel big turbulence on a plane, when I think about earthquakes or worry about another DM flare-up coming. I continually practice tackling my fears by recognizing, acknowledging and rejecting them. I tell myself that fear is only in my head; it has no power over me unless I give it power.

When rejection inevitably comes, I let myself feel the initial disappointment and then go after my dreams with even more determination and passion, as if to show that I won't let fear stand in the way or get the best of me. I remind myself that this is my unique journey, and I shouldn't compare myself with anyone else. I acknowledge that living with a chronic illness has imbued me with special gifts that I alone must use to heal myself and inspire others. I use actions like posting my daily musings as positive affirmations that all is well despite my disability. I created a vision board with words and pictures representing my aspirations, and I look at it daily. I've started telling myself that I'm worthy of success and won't let fear of success get in my way. I've discovered that I've viewed good health and success as mutually exclusive aspirations in which only one or the other is possible. Now I'm visualizing health and success together. I'm not constantly concerned about my disability or obsessing over all the things I can and can't do.

Bottom line: fear no longer stops me from moving forward. I'm learning more each day to trust my path and purpose. Now I view the religion of my youth more as my heritage and less as my spiritual center. I've discovered I believe in God, but not the old, westernized white-male God depicted in the movie *The Ten Commandments*. I believe strongly now that there is energy and light connecting and pervading everything and everyone, similar to "the Force" in *Star Wars*. (I am a child of the seventies, after all!) Rather than finding my temple in a physical institution, I find it in nature, where I can simply observe, recognize, and marvel that I am a part of something bigger than myself, such as the ocean or a mountain or the stars, and let my ego fade into the background. More than anything, I remember I am blessed and surrounded by love, and that makes all the difference in my ability to face my fears head-on and land in a place of faith.

Chapter 5
Following Your Bliss

*"Follow your bliss and the Universe will open doors
where there were only walls."*

—Joseph Campbell, *The Power of Myth*

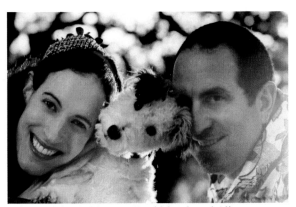

Lisa Sniderman, David Sands and Alice
Credit Jadoo Moments Pet Photography

My name *Lisa* was derived from the Hebrew name Aliza, which means "joyful." It's a very fitting name for me, since joy is not just a feeling I sometimes get, an attitude I adopt, or a mask I put on; it's part of my very core. I often tell people I am happiest and thrive most when I've found and live in my place of joy.

Where I seek or discover joy has changed over the years—from working to protect coastal water quality to hiking, singing, playing guitar and writing songs, creating full-length musicals, or spending quality time with David and Alice, our wire fox terrier. My joy place is where I'm passionate about exploring, learning, discovering, creating, or teaching something.

I remember questioning in 2011 how I was spending my limited energy. A craniosacral therapist came to our house for the first time when my DM was getting worse, and I was experimenting with alternative therapies as well as Western medicine. I told her I'd been expending my limited energy on art and music and asked her, "Is that energy I should be using instead to heal my body?"

She wouldn't even let me finish the question. "Music and art *are* your healing," she declared with authority. It was very affirming.

Acclaimed novelist Alice Walker said, "Whenever you are creating beauty around you, you are restoring your own soul." I live by this adage, spending nearly every waking hour when I'm alone focused on some aspect of music and art. I've come to believe that everything I do is art; it just takes different forms. It isn't so much the medium but the expression and desire to create and connect with myself and others that drives me. It's as if something is compelling me to do it, perhaps my own muse. I believe that when I'm passionate about something like my music and art, I'll find the motivation to make it happen and keep at it. Even when I've been too sick to leave my house or, at times, my bed, expressing myself artistically has been healing.

For example, as I mentioned earlier, while I was recovering from my long hospital stay, I wrote new songs, recorded vocals, made a music video, developed and released a website, started blogging and connecting with new friends and fans online, released a new EP and music video, and called into radio shows for interviews. All from home.

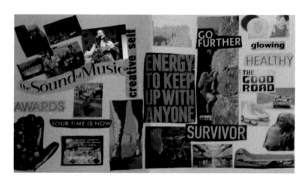

Lisa Sniderman DM Best

I think that artistic expression gives me more than just something to focus on other than being sick. I thrive and experience so much pure joy in the creative process. I'm laser focused and absorbed, and time moves at lightning speed. I live in the moment, in my zone or "flow," and follow my bliss. When I'm excited or passionate about learning and doing something new, I feel more productive, curious, and open to new, outside-the-box ideas, positive energy, and flow. It's as if I'm totally aligned with what inspires me, and I feel fulfilled. I believe I can do anything I set my mind and heart to, and then when I achieve my goal, the cycle continues.

Living with a chronic illness, I need to enter this place of joy often, not just when I'm inspired, but also when days seem their darkest. I know my disease will still be there when I emerge, but for those moments or hours of flow, my ego drops away, my disease disappears, and there is just the joy.

As I've found myself turning more and more to creativity, my curiosity and my analytical mind have led me to explore the link between creativity and healing and the science behind it. Multiple studies show, for example, that nature and works of art boost the immune system.[4] So taking in the beauty and awe of the Grand Canyon, passively listening to a recording of Mozart, or actively working with paint and canvas can actually fight off disease! Apparently, engaging in art can lower levels of chemicals that trigger inflammation and illness. It can even reduce stress, fear, and depression. I loved discovering this. I knew firsthand that when I focused on my art, it would enhance my mood and emotions, but it also means that when I'm walking in nature, exploring and wondering about the world around me, and even just listening to music, I'm actually positively influencing my health. I can heal myself from within!

Perhaps that's why I instinctively turned to singing during my first IVIG infusion treatment in January 2010. I distinctly remember being anxious and fearful going in, half sitting and half lying in that hospital chair with those god-awful fluorescent lights glaring over me from above, and thinking, *Please, God, let me get through this.* It was one of the only times I questioned whether I would make it through the treatment. I needed to know that skilled nurses were standing by, ready to quickly attend to me if anything happened.

Why I was so freaked out, I cannot say. Perhaps it was just the prospect of having something foreign infused in my body that had been extracted from thousands of donors, and not having prior experience with the procedure to feel comfortable or safe. It could have been fear of the unknown or death, or maybe it was hearing the nurse recite the endless list of possible risks and side effects. None of these left me with a warm and fuzzy feeling.

In the midst of my fear, I did the only thing I could think to do: I slowed my breathing, asked for another blanket (which came heated, straight from an oven), and held David's hand. I let myself be in that yucky, medicated space because I knew I had no choice. And then, when my heart was still racing so fast it felt as if it were coming out of my chest, I began to sing. The words just came out. It was the one thing I knew deep inside that would pull me out of that place of fear. I sang the first verse of a new song I had recently written:

If You Already Knew

What if you were born
Knowing how your life would unfold
Where you'd skin your knees
When you'd see your first rainbow
What if you couldn't choose
What you'd say or do
There'd be no surprises or waiting for signs-es
If you already knew[5]

I couldn't have dreamed up more appropriate words to speak to my heart on that occasion. A few nurses even came by to investigate and listen to my voice. All I knew was I had to sing, and I knew then that somehow I would get through this. I knew instinctively that my place of joy inside was where healing would come from.

My creative mind-set has helped me get through other anxiety-producing medical procedures. Having DM has resulted in years of lab work, screenings, and other tests. Sometimes I had diagnostic tests, like X-rays or MRIs. I needed an MRI to assess disease activity and the amount of muscle damage in my arms, and then my legs, when they were becoming weaker.

When I was in the hospital, I had an MRI to help explain why I couldn't move my muscles. MRIs required parts of my body to be strapped down on a moving table, which the technician then slid into a dark tunnel. It was a confining experience, and I had to remain completely still for the whole procedure. If I needed to stop a particular sequence, I could push a button to speak with the technician, who was in a different room. I also wore special goggles that allowed me to see outside the tunnel, even while I was strapped down. As the machine took pictures, it also emitted horrendously loud noises in a predictable pattern directly into my ears through my headphones and even through the earplugs I was wearing to block out some of the sound.

The only thing I could do, on top of taking a sedative to relax me, was to treat every pulse I heard and felt as music, no matter how loud, jarring, long, short, or excruciating it was. No matter how many times the same sound repeated in a sequence, my mind treated it like a rhythmic instrument. It was a drum, and I invented a song right then and there, or sometimes I started singing my own song in my head, using the beat of the pulses. I focused on the music in the vibrations. It was like a song I recorded in 2010 called "Can't

Stop the Music." The idea was that music is everywhere and in everything: alarm clocks, televisions, babbling coffeepots, humming refrigerators, barking dogs, rolling trains, phones, conversations. Every sound can be music, and music is also in me. Hearing music in the incessant clicking noise was the only way I knew to get through the MRIs.

I didn't even realize the significance of music and the role it played in my life until January 2011 when I had an interview with my publicist, and he asked me what my story was. He was looking for an angle he could use in a press release for my upcoming digital EP. All I could offer up were my accolades, or that I had cofounded a women's music-and-art collective called WomenROCK in 2006, or that I had created songs and a story combining my passions for music and water. After mentioning in passing that I wasn't doing live shows at the moment because of some "health" issues, and that I'd been in the hospital in September and was at home recovering now, I suggested that I might be able to perform again in late 2011.

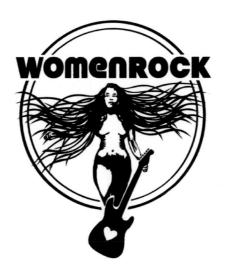

WomenROCK logo—Credit Sylvia Roberts

"No performances? No tours? Where's the story?" my publicist asked. "So you said you were in the hospital for twenty-four days, right?"

"Yeah."

"Wow, people who get heart bypasses are out in just a few days now. And you're releasing an album, retaining PR, releasing a video, and shooting a new one, all while going back and forth for doctors' appointments and infusions and physical therapy and occupational therapy and …?"

I got it. As he asked the questions, I blurted out of nowhere with certainty and passion, "Music is my lifeline!" The tears began to well up and finally spill out because at last I understood what I, Aoede, the Muse of Song, was here to do. I truly got it. I suddenly knew that my story is about persevering through this darkness called DM by engaging in the creative process.

Musician and author Charlie Peacock says, "It's not just about creativity. It's about the person you're becoming while you're creating." For me, creating fosters hope and positivity. I've also discovered that music and art are connecting experiences between listener and artist, and knowing I can connect positively with others through mine also impacts my health. I feel most alive and deeply connected to others when I'm creating and sharing stories and recordings. Ultimately, creating transforms the lens through which I see the world.

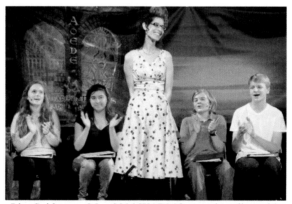

Lisa Sniderman May 2014 WADMO staged reading with
San Carlos Children's Theater San Carlos, CA—Credit Gregg Harris

Chapter 6
Putting Yourself Out There

*"Everyone's journey is unique. Just keep putting yourself out there.
Some will aspire to be where you are; some will be inspired by you;
others will inspire you."*

—Instagram message, TheNotsoSuperMom

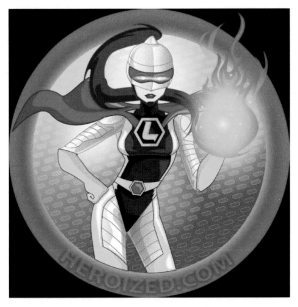

Lisa Hero—Credit heroized.com

As an indie artist with a unique niche—creating full-length fantasy musicals on audiobooks and adapting them to musical-theater stage plays—I have no template to follow. I'm constantly stretching myself and taking risks.

When my muse started to flow in 2002, I didn't question whether I could create music. Of course I would get nervous before performing or wonder and care about how my fans and friends might react to new songs when I played them live or released a new album or musical audiobook. But I've never thought, *I can't do this.* I've always just set my sights on something, worked hard to make it happen, and then put myself out there, diving headfirst into uncharted waters.

I attribute my risk-taking nature and self-assurance in large part to my parents. I've been filled with appreciation, wonder, and curiosity about the world since I was a child. My parents encouraged creativity of all kinds, from drama to singing, playing instruments, dancing, and modeling. They instilled a can-do attitude in me that has helped me navigate the DM diagnosis and living with a chronic illness for more than a decade. Through their words and actions, their constant message has always been, "We believe in you!" which has given me confidence to be and do anything I want, try on different hats, be übercreative, believe in myself, and shine. I've been putting myself out there all my life.

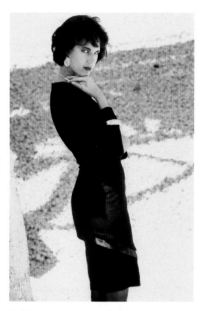

Lisa Sniderman 1986 Modeling in Los Gatos, CA

However, when it came to sharing my health issues, I didn't know how to reconcile my desire to connect with people and present my public face as an artist with my desire to keep my health issues private. As early as January 2009, I struggled with how much to say because I was concerned it could have an impact on my career, especially if another artist, producer, or venue booker were to think, *I won't ask her to do a gig. She's sick and unable to rise to the occasion.* What's wild is when I did go public in February 2011, I attracted people who needed light and hope.

One mother of a child who was struggling with JM wrote:

Thanks for giving us hope that Eldon will also be able to accomplish amazing things in his life. We look forward to seeing all the great things you will continue to do! There are a lot of moms in the support group commending you on your amazing accomplishments, and you have given a lot of moms a lot more optimism for their babies' futures.

Another mother said:

My nine-year-old daughter was diagnosed three years ago with juvenile dermatomyositis, and you have been a big inspiration to her. It's nice for her to see she is not alone. Thank you for being such a positive influence without even knowing the lives you touch.

And a fellow DM sufferer wrote:

It's always good to get the reminder to do "what you can with what you've got" when it feels like so much has been taken away by this disease.

I also put myself out there when dealing with the press. In 2011, in the press release for my digital EP of new Aoede quirky pop songs, the headline read, "Artist Perseveres against Rare and Debilitating Disease While Inspiring Others through Creative Process." There it was, in bold, for the world to see. I didn't want to play the sympathy card, and I wasn't ready to take on that disabled-artist identity. But by giving radio interviews and features over the years and allowing interviewers to decide the content of the health-related questions they asked, I've responded as honestly as I could and have had a positive impact on listeners and readers. I've learned that an important part of my journey is letting go of what others might think and becoming comfortable talking openly about my illness.

Over time I've discovered that I grow as an artist and person when I venture outside my comfort zone and hold on to hope, no matter what. Back in June 2012, when I released my album *Skeletons of the Muse*, I chose to do something I had never done: combine multimedia, including video, readings, and live performance. For the show, I had a full ensemble and was able to just sing without playing guitar. It was very freeing. I'd been confident and strong pre-DM, so I was a little anxious about performing. Pre-DM, I didn't have to think about consistency, whether I would need to sit, or what my energy level would be on show day. But putting on this show—putting myself out there—helped me get over some of this anxiety.

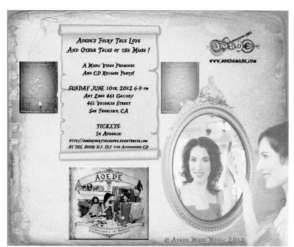

Aoede April 2012 *Fairy Tale Love* music video
and *Skeletons of the Muse* release poster

Also in 2012, as I said earlier, I was particularly challenged and empowered when I decided to try a new direction as an artist and create a musical story. After I received positive feedback from adults and kids alike at my CD-and music-video-release party in June, my producer encouraged me to make a children's album. I had an idea to create a compelling fairy-tale story for tweens that ultimately became my first musical-story audiobook, *Is Love a Fairy Tale?* I wrote new songs for the project, created colorful characters and a fantasy setting, found an amazing illustrator, sang duets, and imagined a whole world of musical stories, complete with narration and magic. I collaborated with my producer on the story, music, and concepts. I had contributions from wonderful voice-over actors and a narrator, as well as stellar musicians. I had never recorded spoken words on an album or had others sing with me, but I welcomed and embraced all of these firsts and really enjoyed writing for young people.

Writing a full script and creating an award-winning children's album, when I'm best known for my pop music, allowed me to grow as an artist. I challenged myself to write for a different audience, which helped me find a new niche and continue creating and recording musicals. I even submitted *Is Love a Fairy Tale?* for consideration for a Grammy Award, though it didn't advance to the nomination stage. None of this would have happened if I hadn't strongly believed in myself and my music and allowed myself to be vulnerable and try something new in a world I was just becoming familiar with.

I continually push myself as an artist, submitting my music and art to contests and competitions and allowing my peers to judge my music, audiobooks, music videos, and stage plays. Knowing that many people could be listening to and judging my music can be intimidating at times, but this has forced me to take the necessary time to create unique, top-notch products.

In 2013, I released my second musical-story audiobook, *What Are Dreams Made Of?* (WADMO), which ended up winning several awards and was also considered for a Grammy Award. Further, I was a finalist and winner in two major songwriting competitions, and several film and TV companies licensed and pitched my music. Receiving nominations and awards in multiple media formats has been incredible not only for validating that I'm on the right path artistically, which drives me to continue pursuing my dreams and increases my confidence, but also for helping me gain recognition and credibility in the industry.

In 2014, I adapted WADMO into a theater production and worked with a children's theater to hold a staged reading of the musical, even though I'd never worked with young actors before or written for the stage. I also signed with an artist management agency for acting and modeling.

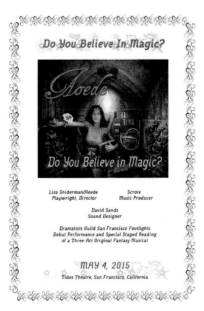

MAGIC May 2015 staged reading program

In 2015, I completed my third musical-story audiobook, *Do You Believe in Magic? (MAGIC)* and submitted it for consideration for a Grammy Award. I successfully completed an advanced-training class for playwrights and performed a monologue, song, and commercial at a talent showcase in Los Angeles (dressing and singing in a fairy-tale costume, complete with tiara, as well as performing in my bathrobe!). I also traveled to a Dramatists' Guild conference and even stayed by myself for a few days. Achieving this level of independence empowered me.

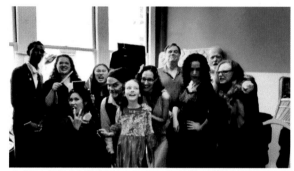

Aoede May 2015 *MAGIC* cast, staged reading Tides Theatre, San Francisco—Credit Christine Kessel

In 2016, I completed voice-over work for a children's audiobook, *The Magic World of Bracken Lea*; taught ten weeks of workshops for young adults; directed staged readings of *MAGIC;* and secured a grant from the National Arts and Disability Center, which funded the creation of instrumental sound tracks from existing recordings that I will use to accompany live performances of *MAGIC.*

The late actor Christopher Reeve once said, "So many of our dreams … at first seem impossible, then they seem improbable, and then, when we summon the will, they soon become inevitable!"[6] I'm living proof of this. Yet even though taking risks and throwing myself at new challenges and opportunities can be rewarding, it doesn't always result in positive outcomes. As Internet entrepreneur Chris Dixon observed, "If you aren't getting rejected on a daily basis, then your goals aren't ambitious enough." I tend to believe it.

Though I've received countless positive messages, awards, reviews, and so much support, I'm always dealing privately with rejections in some aspect of my career, especially with regard to licensing and placing my music, being selected for gigs, being awarded grants, and pitching my musicals to theaters looking to produce new works. I've been told that my grant-application proposals aren't competitive enough; that my original fantasy musicals aren't a good fit for a particular theater or school program; that one of my songs isn't right for a TV show; that my albums didn't advance to the nomination stage. The majority of the time, I never even get a response when I put myself out there. On an online artist platform and gig submission site, for example, I wasn't selected for 84 percent of the opportunities for which I submitted my songs in 2012. (That's sixteen out of nineteen submissions!) But each time I'm rejected, I tell myself I'll be fine and will let it go and move on. I reassure myself that something better is in store. I force myself to work harder, try again, send another e-mail, make another call. I never give up. I tell myself that it isn't about the nomination, the award, or the recognition; it's about the journey and the process of growth and development I go through as an artist and a person.

Of all the ways I put myself out there, sharing my personal struggles is perhaps the most daunting. At times, especially because I'm almost always home, I feel like I'm hiding from the world, playing it safe indoors. Maybe that's why I create light characters, focus on fantasy, and want to connect with my inner child. As I've taken on Aoede the Muse's identity, inspiring others, I'm disinclined to share the scary, icky, fearful, sad, negative feelings—the secret spaces where I've stuffed my skeletons. I tell myself I have to put on a smile and be upbeat, not show weakness or have self-doubt. It's much easier to tell the world that all is beautiful than to admit that living with a chronic illness is harder than anything I've ever faced; that some days it's exhausting to get out of bed, despite my positive attitude and optimism; that I get tired of thinking and talking about being sick, and just plain being sick; that the endless therapies, drug cocktails, and unwanted side effects keep me on a roller coaster; that I resent having precious moments of my life replaced with 156 doctors' appointments; that I wish I had more stamina for being in the world; that I wonder where David's and my relationship would be had I never gotten sick—if he didn't have to do all the shopping, cleaning, cooking, and driving, and we had an equal partnership instead of a caretaker-patient relationship. This is the stuff I used to keep to myself, choosing instead to share the positive accomplishments, the milestones, and the fulfillment of dreams I've decided others want to hear about.

But over the years, I've pushed myself to share my struggles with DM and be vulnerable, which has been positive and healing. In fact, I've discovered I can be the hero of my own story if I set my mind to it. In 2014, I wrote a song called "What Makes a Hero." Though intended for Cure JM kids who are dealing with the same disease I'm battling, I think after so many disappointments and rejections that sometimes cause me to question my path, I needed to write that song to remind myself that I, too, am a warrior.

At first, when I thought of the word hero, I conjured up big-screen movie images of the reluctant Bilbo Baggins, the protagonist of *The Hobbit* who, against all odds and only after every imaginable obstacle was thrown in his path, proved himself a worthy burglar and completed his harrowing quest to reclaim treasure from the treacherous dragon, Smaug. Heroes often have defining character traits and act in predictable ways. We might consider them strong and fearless, but they usually also have some flaw or weakness they must overcome to vanquish their mortal enemies. They often have to confront hard truths about themselves before they can transform from what they are to what they need to be.

I've discovered that being the hero of my own story doesn't mean I have to be larger than life. It can be as simple as shifting my attitude and taking chances despite the obstacles that are thrown in my way. If something scares me, I usually jump at the chance to try it and then immerse myself in it. I embrace new opportunities and dare to dream big. I acknowledge my fears and doubts and then reject them. I don't allow past failures or perceptions of myself as not good enough, strong enough, or worthy enough to dictate my future. I've decided I'm already a hero for battling my illness every day and not letting it define or defeat me. I can also be a hero by inspiring others and giving back, especially to those who are also fighting illness or have lost their inspiration along the way.

It is said that dreams are what the mind conceives, the heart desires, and the soul believes. Whether it's a big possibility like a production opportunity or a film-festival acceptance, or something small like an e-mail from someone new that may open a new door or begin a friendship, *hope* is what motivates me.

When I have setbacks, hope, above all else, carries me through my darkest days of DM and helps me keep my dreams alive. Hope makes all things seem possible, even if only for a short time. Hope is what I hold in my heart when I send a positive message to the Universe and expect something good to happen that might help me advance my dream. And every time the Universe delivers something that makes me question my path, I may ask what the rejections might be telling me and change course, but I don't lose hope. I remind myself that my dreams don't die because of one particular outcome, that everything happens to bring me to the next part of the journey. Most important, I remain tireless, determined, driven, passionate, committed, and interested in growing and challenging myself. I continue to believe, persevere, work hard, be creative, and inspire myself and others. It's a great alternative to focusing on my DM! It isn't as if I'm no longer sick, but putting myself out there, focusing on my creativity and new challenges, and discovering new niches help me thrive despite my disability.

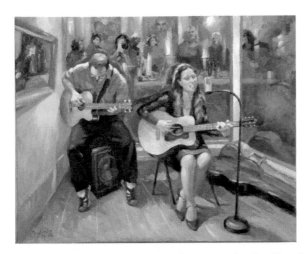

Aoede Apr 2006 SF Women Artists Gallery Reception San Francisco "On The Night of the Reception" Painting—Credit Sandra Lo

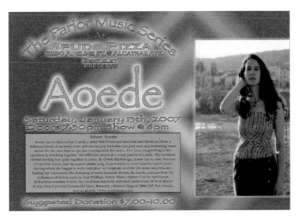

Aoede Jan 2007 performance flyer

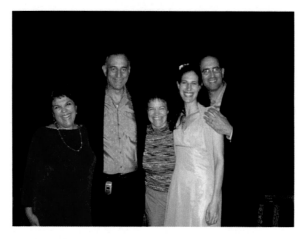

Lisa Sniderman and David Sands May 2008 wedding
reception with Jan, Lou and Debbie Sniderman

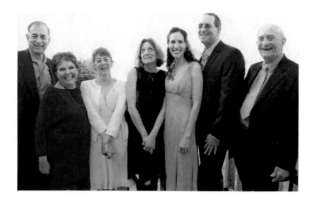

Lisa Sniderman and David Sands May 2008 wedding
reception with Jan, Lou, Helen, Marsha, Sheldon

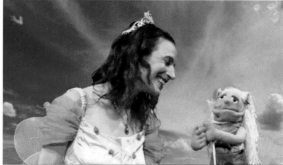

Aoede Apr 2014 Fairy Tale Love by Aoede with Puppets
Credit Uncorked

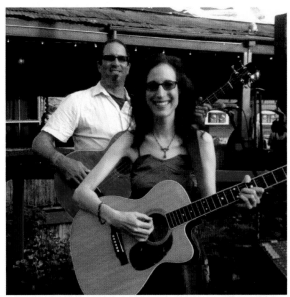

Aoede Apr 2012 IMC Awards House of Blues with David Sands

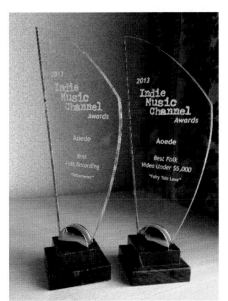 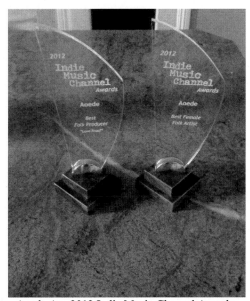

Aoede Apr 2013 Indie Music Channel Awards   Aoede Apr 2012 Indie Music Channel Awards

Chapter 7
Surrounding Yourself With Cheerleaders

"Surround yourself with the dreamers and the doers, the believers and thinkers, but most of all, surround yourself with those who see the greatness within you, even when you don't see it yourself."

—Edmund Lee

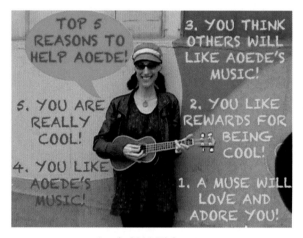

Aoede 2011 Kickstarter

Before the fall of 2010, I was independent. I was no longer driving, but I could walk, dress myself, bathe myself, and eat without help. That all changed once I found myself in the hospital, then rehab, and then home, where I needed assistance to do nearly everything. It wasn't me. I still saw myself as this strong, independent, driven woman, but my body was weak and uncooperative. I couldn't even sit up by myself without becoming exhausted. Part of my journey, I learned, was allowing others to help me, to give me things I needed or do things for me that I could no longer do for myself. It wouldn't be forever, I told myself, and it was a great motivator for recovery because I didn't want to be in a wheelchair and confined to the house. I wanted to have a full life and a real relationship with my husband again!

When I was the sickest and thought about what was most important to me, it was relationships and connections. During my hospital stay and for several weeks afterward, my mom stayed by my side, and then my sister flew in from Florida to help when Mom finally went home to Arizona. Then David's parents arrived from Oregon to step in. David made an online chart where friends could sign up to take me to the hospital and sit with me during my long IVIG treatments, since David had to return to work and couldn't always be there with me for five days each month. I had family and friends around me constantly. They were all very supportive, sharing stories, bringing movies, decorating my room with flowers and cards, and cheering me on in my incremental progress. I felt their love surrounding me and will always be grateful to each of them.

My dad's selfless giving was also so helpful in my recovery and in propelling my dream forward. When I was ready to share my musical-story audiobooks, he spent weeks of his time and energy custom building each of my new album websites. We'd work together, spending hours on the phone creating or placing content or troubleshooting technical issues, and this allowed me not only to spend quality time with Dad but also to focus on something I loved rather than on being sick.

When I joined Twitter in December 2010, it was partly so I wouldn't feel so isolated while I was stuck recovering at home, as well as to find fans and other musicians who might be interested in connecting over music. I began posting my inspirational messages, pictures, questions, wordplays, puns, and other nonpromotional content and building and engaging a whole new fan base of musicians and music lovers. These fans became my virtual cheerleaders. I grew my network from zero to more than twenty-one thousand followers over the next five years!

I didn't understand the implications of having a following until I launched my Kickstarter campaign in late 2011 to fund the release of my album *Skeletons of the Muse*. Seventy-eight generous people contributed more than $5,000 so I could release the album I had recorded. What it meant to me went way beyond being funded, though. It meant that though I was confined to my home, I somehow had an impact on these people by connecting on social networks, building and nurturing relationships, sharing my story and my music, and hearing their stories. Many of my backers were relatives or friends, of course, and I'm ever so grateful for their sweet support. But having total strangers on Facebook and Twitter offer to help me make my music was so unexpected and wonderful.

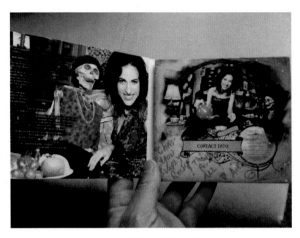

Aoede 2011 Kickstarter

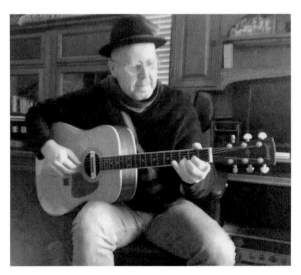

Scrote, Producer, San Mateo, CA

One of the most important things I've learned as a result of having DM is that I don't do life alone. I assembled and surrounded myself with a talented and highly motivated team of people who believe in me. I collaborated on five albums with my amazing producer, Scrote, who helped me implement my visions between 2010 and 2015. I found and worked with a fabulous PR and marketing team that still stays connected to me and supports my dreams. I couldn't have thrived through chronic illness without my incredibly supportive family, the Grammy music community I've built, the friends and fans who respond to my monthly newsletters, and the virtual fans who've engaged with me on social media and my website. All these beautiful cheerleaders offer steadfast support and encouragement, feedback, and love that help me sustain the drive to create, express, and put my music and art out into the Universe. It isn't a one-way street either. When I share some small success, most often others share their stories and successes with me as well.

My husband is my number-one cheerleader. David's parents, and mine, have modeled the value of a lifelong marriage partnership. David's parents just celebrated their sixtieth wedding anniversary, while mine recently celebrated fifty years. With their strong relationships in mind, I took very seriously the first question our rabbi asked David and me as we sought counsel before getting married.

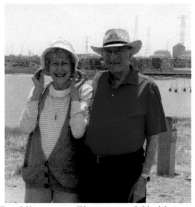 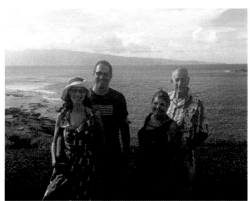

David's parents Florence and Sheldon Slomowitz, San Mateo, CA   Lisa's parents Jan and Lou Sniderman, Sep 2017 50th Anniversary, with David, Maui

"What is the rip in the fabric of the Universe that you two have come together to mend or repair?" This intriguing question gave me goose bumps and immediately piqued my interest in what this strange contemporary reconstructionist rabbi would say next. It was the first time I had considered that beyond our own respective life journeys, there was a special purpose in our union.

We pondered the question silently when he posed it, and over the subsequent weeks, we began to formulate our own responses, which finally made their way into our ketubah, our Jewish marriage contract that spelled out our spiritual vows to each other and our shared responsibilities. We discovered that our purpose together, divinely inspired, was to spread soulfulness, to inspire and effect change around us through our activities and partnership, open communication, and the support of each other's creative growth. We promised to continually invest in our partnership, striving to renew our friendship and our romantic spark each day. Many of our friends have remarked on our solid and loving relationship through our sixteen years together. Some have even told us they wish to follow our example.

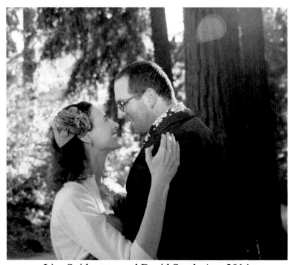

Lisa Sniderman and David Sands Aug 2014
Credit Stephanie Secrest Photography

My first marriage had lasted nearly seven years. We met when I was eighteen and attending UC Santa Barbara. He lived in San Jose and would make the long drive to visit me at UCSB every weekend. I eventually moved back to Northern California in 1992 to attend UC Santa Cruz, and we lived together until we finally married in 1995, when I was twenty-two.

He was a wonderful, devoted man, and my best friend, but over time, we grew apart. We shared a house and bed and friends and families, but no life dreams. As the years progressed, I felt as though we were living separate lives, and I was longing for spiritual connection and communication that I couldn't find in this relationship. Ironically, when I left the marriage in late 2001, it enabled both of us to grow in ways we never could have had we stayed together. I discovered music, embarked on a path of discovery, and found my voice and my muse. My ex-husband, I learned, pushed himself harder than ever and discovered competitive cycling and surfing. Sometimes letting go and moving on is the only way we grow.

When I met David in September 2002, I wasn't looking for a long-term relationship, least of all another marriage. I was casually dating a few people, and my divorce wasn't even final until October. Apparently, David wasn't looking for a serious relationship either, since he'd also been married—twice—and divorced. A friend of ours introduced us, claiming he was playing matchmaker. We both like to think he takes credit for the match only because David and I hit it off!

Perhaps prophetically, David and I connected over music. I was returning a CD to our matchmaking friend, Robert, a singer in a local alternative-rock band whom I had met and befriended on a commuter train. David, who used to play bass in Robert's band, was hanging out at Robert's house when I showed up to return the CD, and Robert invited us both to dinner.

David was easy to talk to, and eventually we found we could talk about anything and everything for hours and never tire of each other. David was much older than me, and I initially saw him as a friend, not a love interest. He was close to my age now when I met him. I was twenty-nine. But there was an ease and comfort I enjoyed around him, and no pressure to be anything, which allowed our friendship to develop over several months instead of being based on attraction like so many of the relationships with other men I had dated.

I remember how David lit up when he drove me around San Francisco pointing out all the houses with really cool artsy gates. He had a metal shop, and I learned early on how much art and creativity sparked him. He encouraged me to pursue singing in a cover band, even letting me rehearse with him. I discovered that David had played bass since he was fifteen years old and loved music, performing in as many projects as he could. I found in David qualities and attributes I didn't even know I was seeking: he was a soul mate, a thinker, a musician and artist, and a patient teacher eager to share his vast knowledge about everything with me, who never stopped asking questions. A true Renaissance man, he could speak Cantonese, ski, play bass, fix or build anything electronic or mechanical, and create beautiful metal art. The world filled us both with a wild curiosity and wonder, and he'd had experiences I only dreamed about.

We'd been together just under five years when David returned from his fifth trip to China for work, including a stopover in Singapore, and presented me with a beautiful engagement ring, thoughtfully sized so I could still play my guitar and not worry about damaging it. He proposed in 2007 at our favorite little local restaurant in San Francisco, adding that he didn't want to spend any more time on trips without me. He likes to point out that I was oblivious to the lead-up to his proposal because I kept changing the subject or looking at the menu. But this man had won my heart five years earlier, and I couldn't even imagine spending life without him either. So without hesitation, I said "Yes!" and amid tears and cheering and clapping in the restaurant, he placed on my finger the diamond ring he had carried so many miles.

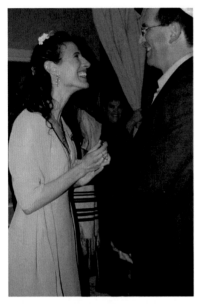 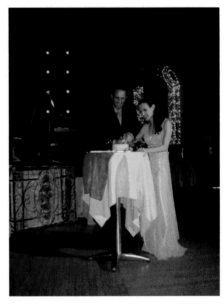

Lisa and David May 2008 wedding, Jenner, CA, and wedding reception in San Francisco

I was diagnosed with DM less than a year later, six weeks before our spring wedding, which, because of our love of music, we decided to make a joint reception and CD-release party for my first full-length album *Push and Pull*. I remember asking David just after being diagnosed if he still wanted to marry me, considering I had just learned I had a rare autoimmune disease and an uncertain future. He said of course, that it changed nothing for him or the way he felt about me.

It has turned out that our entire married life has revolved around living with DM: with me as the patient and him as the caretaker. I doubt that either of us realized what a life with DM would be like, and neither of us was prepared for the unexpected flare-up of my DM in 2010 that rendered me completely helpless for months.

How do you prepare yourself, let alone a marriage, for an event like that? I learned during those difficult weeks of hospitalization and months of recovery just what kind of partner I had in David. He came to visit me in the hospital every day, and when I was finally ready to go home, he built a ramp outside for my wheelchair and readied the house with a raised toilet seat, shower chair, indoor ramps over our steps, and everything else he could think of to make the transition easier.

Throughout the six months of IVIG infusions, he took off work as often as he could to sit with me through the five-hour treatments for five days each month. He would work full days and then come home to cook, clean, and shop. He would prepare all our meals, and because I had difficulty swallowing, he would even cook turkey for me and then lovingly grind it up in the blender so it was soft enough for me to swallow. Even today, he still does all the driving and most of the housework, shopping, and cooking—all with a full-time job!

He's never looked at me differently despite my wheelchair, or my walker and cane. He views these only as tools to help me and continues to see me, not my disability. I've considered it a huge burden for him to carry my wheelchair, help me with almost everything, and drive me everywhere. But he's told me that giving makes him feel good, and that my gratitude, love, appreciation, and positive attitude make him want to help me even more.

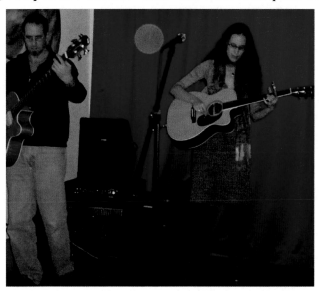

Aoede Nov 2007 with David Sands

David has also supported my creative spark since the onset of DM. He and I played together for years in Aoede, as a duo since 2006, and as a band with our drummer, John, from 2007–2009. He has also been an integral part of all my Aoede projects, from recording my vocals to playing stand-up bass and percussive metal, carrying my guitars and setting up the sound at our shows, helping make each of the studio days easier on me, and doing full sound reinforcement at my musical-theater shows. He also accompanied me to every awards show in Los Angeles, driving us down from San Francisco, and always cheered loudly as Aoede's name was called for an award, after which he would pick me up and lovingly carry me to the car or hotel room so I could rest.

David has been instrumental in shaping my attitude, my passion and drive for art and music, and my recovery. I wouldn't be the person I am today without him by my side, encouraging, supporting, enabling, and loving me without condition. He gives me so many reasons to get up each morning. He's a saint, and I'm blessed beyond measure to have him as my life partner.

In 2009, I wrote a special song for David's fiftieth birthday and sang it to him in front of all our friends.

50 Things I Fell in Love With

1. You own a pink manly telephone but
2. You curse your Bluetooth just like blue Volvos
3. You hold me tight when I'm scared
4. You play with my short, curly hair
5. You laugh at dinosaurs with tiny arms
6. You take me on picnics in our little park
7. You drop me off and park the car
8. You've tried most everything so far
9. You don't think you can bow a bass
10. You teach me something new every day
11. You heavy lift around our house
12. You shake me, pick me from our couch
13. You rescue all of those who ask and
14. You never, never wear a mask
15. You fall asleep at my feet
16. You're just you in front of me-ee-ee

50 things I've longed to tell you
50 perfect little truths
50 things I fell in love with … You

17. You use soup as your Facebook face
18. You say Shallow Alto and San Jose-B
19. You bought me a bike and an amp and

20. You sacrifice so I can nap
21. You are kind to our families
22. You're talented beyond belief
23. You fix or build a mean machine
24. You can order in Chinese
25. You drive shiny electric cars
26. You're always carrying my guitars
27. You pull on gray fleece every day
28. You never judge what people say
29. You scream at spiders and blue Volvos but
30. You took that dead mouse out before I woke
31. You built us a chuppah for two
32. You said, yes, I do-oo-oo

50 things I've longed to tell you
50 perfect little truths
50 things I fell in love with …

33. You-oo-oo-oo-you dare to dream and
34. You-oo-oo-oo-you fell for me
35. You call me and you make me smile
36. You play your bass with lots of style
37. You love your bear and benda toys
38. You're not like other boys
39. You pour your heart into boats and dreams
40. You write me notes and take care of me
41. You sing along with '70s songs
42. You play with frogs and poo dogs
43. You fry pasta with ketchup to eat
44. You'll never run out of curiosity
45. You're a history whiz and
46. You own a cool metal biz
47. You put others in front of you but
48. You pour toxic mold so I don't have to
49. You work on Poor Blue for me
50. You sometimes let me heat seek
50 things I've longed to tell you
50 perfect little truths
50 things I fell in love with …

You-oo-oo-oo-oo-oo-oo-oo-oo

Oh you-oo-oo-oo I fell for you
Talkin' 'bout
You-oo-oo-oo-oo-oo-oo-oo-oo-oo-oo
Birthday boy
You-oo-oo-oo-oo-oo-oo-oo-oo-oo
50 things I'm still in love with ... You[7]

Living well with a chronic illness requires physical, emotional, and spiritual support, and I'm so fortunate to have it in such abundance. But no one cheers for me as loudly and consistently as David does, and through the years, I continue to find more things in him to fall in love with.

Chapter 8

Finding Positive Role Models

"Be strong. You never know who you are inspiring."

—Unknown

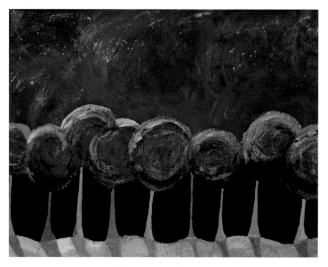

Trees at Night—Credit Amberlin Wu

One of the most positive things I've done as I've learned to live with my disability is to seek out others who have been through what I'm going through and can serve as role models, offering insight and wisdom from their own experiences. Sometimes just connecting with someone who also has a chronic illness and understands without my having to explain can be so affirming.

When I think of amazing role models I've had throughout my illness, both my mother-in-law and my mom immediately come to mind. David's mom, Florence, has been living with lupus for many years and is almost eighty-two. She has shown me time and again, through her words and actions, that she doesn't let lupus rule her life, despite her fatigue, pain, skin rashes, flare-ups, and other persistent aches and ailments. Though she receives monthly infusions and has immunosuppressive treatments, I rarely hear her talk or complain about her disease. She is always more concerned with how David and I, and my parents, are feeling than how she might be faring. Her general attitude seems to be "Accept the hand life has dealt you, but seize the moment now, while you still can." She is always giving thoughtful, heartfelt gifts and doing little things for family and friends to show her love, like baking me special gluten-free, sugar-free brownies or getting up early to make bag lunches from scratch for all her "kids" for our long drives home over the holidays.

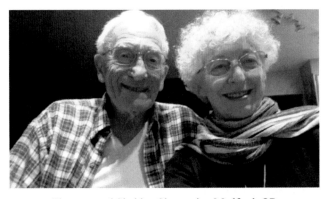

Florence and Sheldon Slomowitz, Medford, OR

Florence and I have shared many of the same symptoms and treatments over the years. I'm so fortunate to have someone in my life who gets what I'm going through and is so filled with genuine concern and love. Over the course of my treatment, Florence has helped me become less anxious each time I've been given a new drug. I've seen how she simply accepts each treatment as the one that could help her better manage or even improve her quality of life, or help her pain, and she doesn't let all the risks or possible horrific side effects paralyze her. If she has fear or anxiety about her treatments, she hides it well. She has shown me that although she has a chronic illness, she won't let it stop her from doing the things she loves.

She and Sheldon, David's eighty-eight-year-old dad, continue to live rich, active lives, filled with close, warm, supportive friendships, frequent social and family events, a ton of cooking and baking, volunteer work, classes, and even long road trips and new adventures together. All of her life lessons have been instrumental for me in learning how to live in harmony with, and not fight against, my own illness.

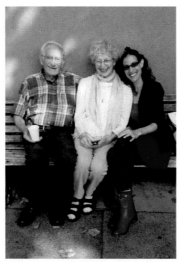

Florence and Sheldon Slomowitz
with Lisa Sniderman, San Mateo, CA

My parents, too, have always been positive role models through their actions, values, and behavior, even before I knew what a role model was. But my mom is the one who not only helped me through the worst of my DM by being with me throughout the entire hospital stay and my rehabilitation at home, but also continues to show by example how to live with chronic illness day in and day out. My mom has been through more than her share of autoimmune diseases, hospital stays, and lengthy treatments and infusions, but to add icing to the cake, she's been battling continual shoulder injuries that have necessitated upwards of fourteen surgeries to repair the damage.

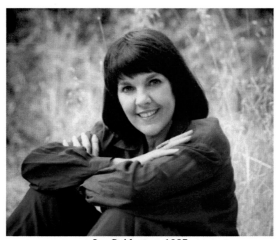

Jan Sniderman 1987

Regardless of the fatigue, ailments, pain, or affliction she is enduring at the moment, I see Mom soldier on through it all. Unless someone brings up her health and asks her directly, I don't hear her complain about the hand life has dealt her. She goes about her life the best she can, cheerfully, with love and gratitude and a positive attitude. I believe she has also learned she has limitations, respects her body's need to rest, and doesn't push herself too much. I see her focus on what she can do, not on what she can no longer do. She gives willingly of her valuable time and limited energy to others, such as helping me with research on the latest treatments for DM or coming with me to the practitioner's office when I was exploring alternative therapies.

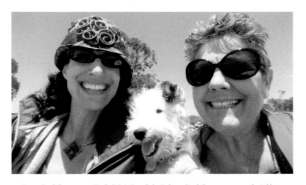

Jan Sniderman Jul 2015 with Lisa Sniderman and Alice

As a former librarian, she loves collecting, sorting, and sharing information, and she's a ravenous reader. My mom is always sending me health-related articles, positive quotes, and funny dog-related or inspirational videos and stories, driven by her love and compassion and her genuine desire to see me healed—or at least have the best quality of life I can, given what I've been dealt. It's also a great comfort to me to know I can and do talk to Mom, and she'll get what I'm going through. Sometimes she and I are so in sync that we experience the same symptoms. I don't know whether I inherited my tendency toward autoimmune disease from her, but at least we can navigate the storms together.

The other beautiful role model in my family was my grandma. I believe it's because of her that I look at life and ask, "What can I learn?" or "What can I teach?" By just quietly observing her in 2012, when David and I visited her for her ninety-fifth birthday, I was fortunate to catch a glimpse of the lens through which she saw the world. I watched her sit by the window and gaze at the birds outside with such awe and wonder. I watched her lovingly pet the dogs and feed them scraps. I watched her face light up as Grandma, Mom, and I—three generations—went to the Handicapables therapy class at the swimming pool. I watched her sit outside in the warm sun totally engrossed in her book. I watched her zoom out of the car in her walker, faster than Mom or me, or try to be the first at the restaurant to pay the bill, concealing her credit card in her sleeve, as if we wouldn't notice. I watched as she lit up a room when she walked in, and others couldn't help but be affected by her joy and her light. I watched as she would get dressed up and then ask each day when she could take us to lunch or dinner because she wanted to spend her time out in the world at restaurants with people and good food. I watched as we left the sneak preview at the theater, and she said, "Well, they can't all be winners now, can they?" I watched as she and Mom wrote out, addressed, and sent each thank-you card the day after her birthday. I watched her eyes light up as she listened to me play ukulele and sing her a special birthday song.

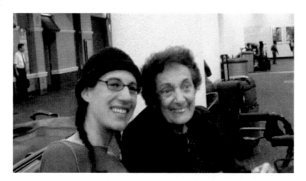

Lisa and Grandma Mar 2009 Bahamas

Grandma embodied beauty, grace, and love and was a role model to me without ever knowing it. I'm sure many of her little gems have helped me navigate my life and my illness. She left this earth in 2015, but her light continues to shine in everyone she touched, and in me. Here are some of the life lessons I learned from watching her:

1. Embrace each new day with love, wonder, and gratitude.

2. Treat all creatures (especially dogs and birds) with kindness and love and make them feel special.

3. Spend time each day just observing nature and beauty.

4. Recognize everything in life as a gift. Acknowledge and appreciate the little things and feel blessed to receive each one.

5. Give in every way you can to everyone you can.

6. Have a positive attitude about your life.

7. Read and keep your mind active. Keep learning and growing.

8. Keep your body active and keep challenging yourself.

9. Focus on the joy, wonder, beauty, and light in all things.

10. Dress up, eat good food, and enjoy good living while you can.

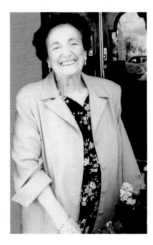

Grandma Rachel Goldman 2005

Another powerful role model for me was a dear childhood friend, Amberlin. We became friends in sixth grade when my family moved from Arizona to California, and we continued to go to school together until we graduated high school.

Starting in her twenties, Amberlin fought tirelessly and courageously for fifteen years against what some consider an invisible disease, chronic fatigue syndrome (CFS) or myalgic encephalomyelitis (ME). She passed away in 2011 at the age of thirty-nine from her debilitation and the complications of CFS. This disease wasn't invisible to her. She lived daily with constant reminders. She regularly posted on her blog and Facebook page information about CFS to educate others and raise awareness of a disease that is often misunderstood. When she wasn't fighting her own disabilities, she turned to art. She painted, made jewelry, and surrounded herself with things she loved, like chickens and nature. She was a light in her community and to all those she touched. A few years ago I purchased a "Be a Light" T-shirt to support her and CFS. I saw that despite her struggles, she strived for the best possible quality of life and was a light in the darkness for so many she met along her life path.

For me, Amberlin represented hope. While she was alive, there was just that much more hope of finding a cure for CFS, hope for her to live in peace with her disease instead of fighting for her life. She inspired me because if she could fight so courageously for so many years while she was struggling and in pain, and if she could raise awareness, connect with others in her community, and make art while she was in and out of hospitals having treatments and trials, then so could I. There was hope for me in dealing with a rare chronic disease too.

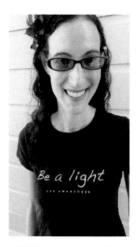

CFS Awareness t-shirt

Her passing didn't extinguish the light. I believe her light shines brighter and brighter each time her story is told, for her message in life—"Be a light"—will continue to spread. It already has. It's become my life purpose.

Chapter 9
Celebrating Your Abundance

"The longer I live the more convinced I become that life is 10 percent what happens to us and 90 percent how we respond to it."

—Charles Swindoll, *Attitudes*

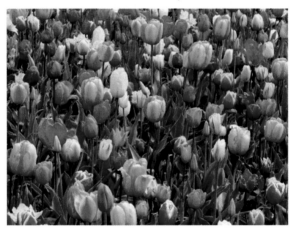

E ven though we can't control what life throws at us, such as a chronic illness, we can control our actions and reactions. I've always believed that. So many times during my illness and career, it would have been much easier to just give up, play the victim, be bitter that my life didn't turn out as I planned, take myriad disappointments and rejections to heart, and not be accountable or take responsibility for the direction and quality of my life. But I never did. Instead, I filled myself with love, gratitude, and a positive attitude, channeled any energy I could muster, and dreamed even bigger. That mind-set has always seen me through whatever life has brought my way.

There have been so many points in my journey when I could have let DM win. For instance, the first time I was administered IVIG, I was anxious and fearful, yet on the morning of the first day of infusions, I posted on Facebook, "I will embrace the day with love and gratitude and a positive attitude." I also found it amazing that we have the technology to create such medicine. I felt blessed and fortunate to have health insurance and be on the receiving end of a product that costs many thousands of dollars. I thought that maybe this was just the treatment my body needed to produce new antibodies, boost my immunity, and kick my DM to the curb.

I wouldn't say that IVIG and I became fast friends, but at least I was learning what to expect each month and was less anxious. I felt blessed to have family or friends take me to the infusion center and sit with me for hours each day as this strange substance fused with proteins in my blood. The infusions took a lot out of my body, and during the week I'd have massive headaches, weight loss from a lack of appetite, brain fog, severe exhaustion, and a hot hand (presumably from the infusion), but I kept soldiering on. I truly believe it makes a difference in the efficacy of treatment if you go into it with a positive attitude. During treatments I imagined all the new antibodies having stories and lives of their own, bursting with health and wellness, strong, eager, and able to kick out all my sick antibodies! I'd like to believe that the treatments, and my attitude that the treatments would work, helped me get better.

To get my head out of sick mode, I would turn to my music, focusing on what brought me joy. In January 2011, I took a six-week interactive online course called The Science of Switching On, taught by an esteemed voice and performance coach, to help me get over my fear of performing in public again. My last performance was in late August 2010, just before my DM flare-up, and when I signed up for the course, I had just spent three months in therapy relearning how to sit up unassisted; stand on my own without holding on to something for balance; walk with a walker, then a cane, and then unassisted; hold and play a guitar; and even sing again after my core muscles had become so weak. Before DM, I couldn't imagine not having the strength to sing. There were times I was nervous before a big show or struggled with getting the right vocal take during a recording session, but I was confident I would access the part of me that wanted to sing. But in 2011, I didn't feel sure about my voice, or even my identity. Would I still be able to sing the way I sang before the flare-up? Could I still connect with my audience? What if I stayed sick? How could I regain my confidence?

Once I began the course, I retained as much as I was able, but I was so exhausted during my infusion weeks that I had a hard time concentrating, which, combined with my core weakness, meant I couldn't even sit through the lectures. I had to explain to the coach why I wasn't able to fully participate—that in addition to the infusions, I was still recovering and undergoing intensive physical therapy. The reality was that I was months away from singing in public. Looking back, I find it amazing that instead of feeling sorry for myself, I kept doing everything I could to prepare myself mentally and physically to perform again.

During that time I also began blogging monthly about being a singer-songwriter living with a disability. I have always loved writing. I kept journals for most of my life, and still do. I excelled in classes like English and journalism in high school and even considered a career in journalism at one time. I found writing essays to be my strong suit in all my classes, especially compared to the confining, ever-tricky multiple-choice-style tests. Give me a one-sentence biology exam question like "Describe DNA and RNA," and I was over the moon and could fill entire blue books.

In college at UC Santa Barbara, I earned an A-plus in a Chicano Studies comparative-literature class that had nothing to do with my declared biology major. I took it to satisfy a requirement and learned I actually had a talent for analytical writing. Perhaps that insight, as well as my barely passing grades in chemistry, led me to switch to environmental studies and eventually focus on environmental law and policy. My love for writing in an unconfined style is why blogging appealed to me when I was just starting to get some focus and concentration back after my hospitalization.

I think I also needed to write to process the roller coaster my mind and body had ridden since the onset of my DM in 2008. Writing about events that transpired allowed me to admit they happened and empowered me to take ownership of them so I could feel some sense of control over how I responded, or better understand when I had to surrender control. Having a chronic illness like DM, where so much is out of my control, has made me realize how I need to be in command of other aspects of my life. It's as if I've replaced my inability to physically drive anymore with ways I can still be in the driver's seat. Blogging also gave some of my fans and friends a glimpse into my private life by helping them understand what DM is and how it has affected me. Further, it allowed me to connect with others who also have DM or another chronic illness and find mutual support. When someone left a comment on one of my blog posts, I would respond, which often led to an unexpected friendship.

It's said that what you focus on expands. I tell myself I have more than enough. I welcome love, good health, strength, stamina, energy, success, and happiness into my life and tell myself I'm worthy. I'm certain that my mental state is tied to my body's well-being. I keep my spirits high and fill my head and heart with love, gratitude, humor, and a positive attitude. This has carried me through the darkness of my DM: depletion, weakness, infections, rashes, fear, anxiety, brain fog, hospitals, and risky experimental treatments. I've learned to keep my focus on what I have instead of what I don't have. And that inevitably leads me to a deep appreciation of my abundance!

Abundance is defined, in part, as "overflowing fullness." This perfectly describes my attitude toward my life. Every day I strive to think, say, and truly believe how blessed I am to live in my place of joy and how grateful I am for all of life's little gifts. I've learned to appreciate and be grateful for all the steps I've taken, no matter how large or small, to improve my strength, health, independence, and quality of life. When I go to bustling, stimulating places like a museum, which I still do with the help of my walker, I wish I had more energy and stamina to stay longer, but I look back and remember it wasn't that long ago when I couldn't do activities for even two hours at a time without becoming exhausted.

While in the rehabilitation hospital, I received an unexpected lesson that helped me see just how blessed I was. It involved watching people much worse off than I. I confess, I wasn't ready to take on others' suffering. It was enough that I had my own experience to deal with. I figured I was learning enough life lessons going through my own ordeal with the goals of getting stronger, not giving up, not losing hope, keeping my positive attitude, having gratitude and love, and feeling blessed. So why did I also have to see the struggles of others less fortunate than I, at least in my eyes?

When I first got to rehab, I saw people who couldn't feed themselves, people who were partially paralyzed, people with speech impediments from strokes, people who lived with constant pain, people who struggled to find words, people who couldn't go to the bathroom without assistance from machines, and people who were incontinent. When I looked at myself, it's no wonder I felt blessed. I saw my situation as temporary. *I will be out of that wheelchair*, I told myself. I could feed myself; I could get to the bathroom with help from my wheelchair; I could speak and think and express myself in words!

The first time I went to group occupational therapy, I felt as if I didn't belong there among the stroke victims, the people who could only partially talk or move, and those I labeled less fortunate. And yet there I was, right next to them, sitting in my wheelchair, relearning the same things they were relearning. Over time I began to see them as people like me, with stories, dreams, hopes, and victories, too. I watched people who looked like me progress incrementally, just like me. They didn't ask to experience strokes or accidents or medical problems that changed their lives in an instant, just as I hadn't expected the changes in my life. Most of these people were courageous, spirited, and driven to do the rehab work. I not only learned empathy and compassion for others I considered less fortunate, but this experience also taught me so much about myself.

We all have difficult things to deal with, and usually when we meet others and learn of their plight, it puts our own "stuff" in perspective. At least, that's my experience. It reminds me of the old proverb, "I felt sorry for myself because I had no shoes—until I met a man who had no feet." My experience also reminds me to accept where I'm at in life and always contrast it with something that could be much worse: I'd rather be home than in the hospital, or when in the hospital, I'd rather be there than not here at all.

Perhaps because I've spent so much time at home, I really value time now. I spend it writing, reflecting, or connecting with others online; playing my guitar or uke; watching shows or movies with David; playing with Alice, our fox terrier; or finding little things that make me laugh. I've replaced *go* and *do* and *see* with a slower, steadier routine. Each day is a true gift that's entirely my own. I treasure this gift over most everything. When I do go outside, it may sound cliché, but the sun is brighter than I remember. The trees are greener. The sky is dotted with cotton balls. I've learned not to take the world around me for granted but to do what Grandma would do and observe nature and each moment with awe and wonder; focus on the joy, wonder, beauty, and light in all things; and acknowledge, accept, and appreciate life's little gifts.

I've discovered that I need to remind myself of my abundance, especially right after a major disappointment or rejection, or when I've had a setback with DM. In those moments, I need to ground myself and tap into the motivation to keep going. For example, I had really wanted, worked hard for, and even expected a particular theater residency. I viewed it as an opportunity of a lifetime to self-produce my musical, with mentorship and funding from a theater company. Convinced this opportunity was custom created just for me, I submitted a well-crafted, thorough proposal. When I received an e-mail informing me that my project hadn't been chosen, I was extremely disappointed and discouraged. I was hoping this particular path was the next one, because opportunities to produce my own show were almost nonexistent. After receiving so much recognition and positive feedback regarding my music, I felt dejected.

But after being knocked down, I got up again. I told myself that something better was coming. I listed all the positives that came out of simply applying for the opportunity, like networking and assembling my creative team and refining my vision. I focused on all I already had—the love of friends, the unconditional support of family, the privilege of spending my days doing what brings me joy, and what I'd gained.

A fan once reached out to me on Twitter, conveying that his wife had lupus and sympathizing with my condition. He asked, "What is the secret to getting beyond a chronic disease?"

"Wow. That's the $100,000,000 question," I told him.

I didn't and don't claim to have the answer to that question. In fact, I have more questions than answers most of the time. But I did share with him some of the things I do when I feel as if everything I'm enduring is too much emotionally, or when I'm so tired of being sick that I feel like staying in bed and shutting the world out:

1. I awaken and greet each day with love, gratitude, and a positive attitude, keeping my spirits high and always having hope.
2. I strive to get the best quality of life I can from each day. I "do what I can with what I've got." I've found peace with a new baseline and a slower pace.
3. I live in my place of joy.
4. I am constantly believing in and telling myself "I am blessed" and "Life is beautiful."
5. I don't do this alone! I recognize when I need help, and I've learned to receive and nurture relationships more than I ever did before. I have an amazing support system; a beautiful, loving family; friends; and a whole network of connections.
6. I make time and find opportunities to create and express myself through art and music.
7. I write to process, share, connect, and inspire others.
8. I play, use humor, and find ways to smile and laugh (and make others smile and laugh) constantly.
9. I affirm the law of attraction and believe I have the ability to attract what is good and positive into my life.
10. I try not to put my limited energy into being, acting, and staying sick. I ask, "What can I give, what can I learn from this, and what can I teach?" not "Why me?" I refuse to be a victim. I am not the disease!

It's not that the illness disappears. I know that some days I'll feel weak and depleted, and rest won't be restorative, but my mind can focus on my place of joy, which helps me heal emotionally and physically. Though my body may have other plans, my spirit and I will keep making music and art, baring what's in my soul, using it to inspire and connect with others, and celebrating my abundance. One day I hope I'll kick this DM to the curb. Until then, I have to settle for kicking the self-pity.

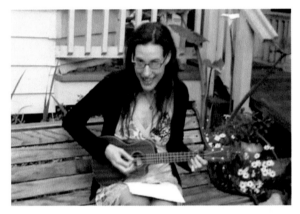

Lisa 2013 playing uke at home, San Francisco

Chapter 10
Keeping Your Dreams Alive

[Stay] strong, confident, and happy—no matter how much
you-gotta-be-friggin'-kidding-me! life throws at you!

—Karen Salmansohn, *Think Happy*

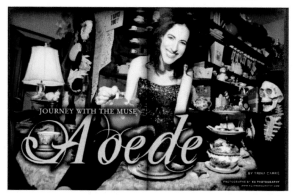

Aoede Aug 2012 online magazine feature Fourculture-issue two

From the moment I was diagnosed with DM, I've watched my chameleon-like dreams shift repeatedly. I let go of some dreams, like playing Caesars Palace or opening for a national act on tour, because I was too sick to chase them. In their place, new dreams were born that I've pursued with drive and passion even while living with DM. Former professional boxer Mike Tyson once said, "I'm a dreamer. I have to dream and reach for the stars, and if I miss a star then I grab a handful of clouds."[8]

I'm a dreamer too. I've come to terms with not being a cookie-cutter mold of an artist. Unlike most artists who release albums and tour to promote them, I haven't been able to perform a full set live, or tour, because of my DM. I call into radio shows for interviews and do online features on my schedule instead of doing personal appearances. I connect and engage with my fans mostly online through social networking rather than in person at shows. I write my musicals and record my own vocals from home with David's engineering assistance. Even while I was collaborating with my producer on all three of my musicals, he always accommodated me and opted for us to do sessions at my house because he knew how much energy was required for me to travel and be "on" for hours at a time.

I measure my progress by what I can realistically accomplish, not by what I'd love to accomplish if I had no limitations. The questions I never stop asking are "How do I keep my dreams alive? What am I capable of? What can I continue to do? And if I can't, what else might I be able to do so I can keep pursuing my dreams?"

I've learned that my goals change from year to year in part because of my waxing and waning energy and also because of my interest in new art forms. Back in 2012, when I began writing the musicals, I recorded on audiobooks, it was a way to keep being a songwriter and share my brand of quirky folk pop with young adults. Several years up the road, I discovered that I also enjoy and have a talent for sharing my vision and working with others to implement it.

Since my primary hats have been singer-songwriter, performer, and recording artist, I had never taught others before March 2015. As a disabled artist at home, I never expected to teach, let alone love doing it. But after my staged reading of WADMO in 2014 and seeing the kind of impact a new musical had on the kids, it got me thinking that I would love to do a school program or workshop to introduce kids to a new musical with the playwright there in the room with them. Maybe it would inspire them to create and write their own works, learn more about the process of writing a play and music from the spark of an idea to completion, and give them experience in staged reading.

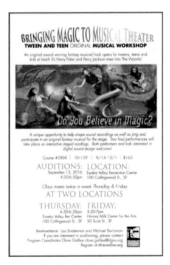 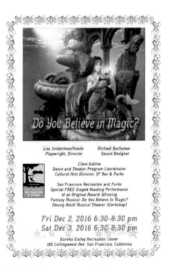

Aoede 2016 Bringing MAGIC to Musical Theater workshop program

I discovered a small local high school for students with learning differences and realized that I wanted to bring these kids a unique workshop experience. So I reached out and actually got a response! The school wanted to start up an afterschool drama class one day a week for two hours, and they needed a teacher. Despite not working outside my house in years, I committed to doing it.

I expected to use my musical as the basis for the class, even perform some of it if there was time. But I threw out my lesson plan once I met with the kids. Most were at a fifth-grade reading level even though they were high school students. I decided it wasn't about me and my agenda, so I gave them a survey asking about their interest areas and then crafted lesson plans designed around these interests to get them excited about theater, work on boosting their confidence, and get them acting, playing, and inspired. Even though it required a ton of energy to keep eight girls with unique needs focused, I learned so much, and later on I ended up incorporating my prep work, games, and modules into a ten-week original musical-theater workshop, which I taught in the fall of 2016. I needed this teaching experience to move me toward what was next. At the time, I had no idea I was planting seeds for future dreams and would gain a whole new joy from working with teens.

If I hadn't allowed my dreams to shift, I might never have found my niche and voice in the world of original musical theater, much less teaching others about my art. In theater I could be the artist in a whole new way. It was still my musical, but I didn't have to be center stage as I did in my recordings. It was freeing to produce and direct workshops and staged readings with musical-theater actors, discover what actors would bring to their characters that wasn't in the script, and see my art through their eyes. Embarking on this new path has also helped me gain more insight into what motivates me most: telling stories.

I keep my dreams alive by first believing in them absolutely and without question, and then I dare myself to fulfill them, even if I don't know how I'll do it. I throw my passion, blood, sweat, tears, and heart into them relentlessly and get lost in their magic until they're realized. I'm a firm believer in the law of attraction. I attract and bring about what I focus on intently, am excited and passionate about, think about incessantly, light up when I talk about, or set in motion. When I dream up powerful, vivid dreams and start taking steps to realize them, the Universe conspires to help me fulfill them.

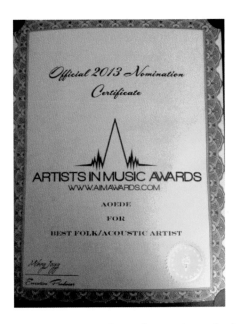

Aoede Dec 2012 Artists in Music Awards nomination

For example, when I entered the Artists in Music Awards in 2012, one of my first post-DM online competitions, I had no idea that Aoede would be nominated for three music awards and would receive two, but I had set something in motion. I believed in my music and my dream, took steps to realize that dream by asking my musical peers for their support, and received more than I ever imagined. Not only did this encourage me to submit songs to other highly competitive international awards programs, but it also publicly validated my music in the industry and gave me confidence to keep dreaming.

When I first was developing my second musical, WADMO, in early 2013, I didn't know how I would realize the vision for the music I heard in my head, let alone the lyrics, melodies, and script I was still writing. I thought maybe my producer, Scrote, and I would gather a few musicians we knew to come record parts at my house. Then in May, we had an opportunity of a lifetime to record the music at the world-famous Ocean Way Recording Studios in Los Angeles, which legends like Frank Sinatra, Michael Jackson, Madonna, Bonnie Raitt, Green Day, and Ray Charles have graced with their presence. It was magical, exactly what my dreams were made of!

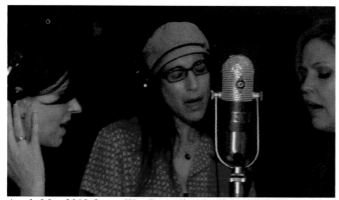

Aoede May 2013 Ocean Way Recording Studios with Holly, Nicki
Los Angeles, CA—Credit Christopher Ewing

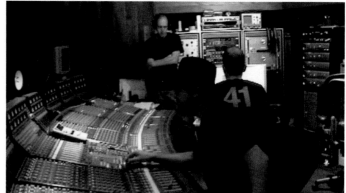

Aoede May 2013 Ocean Way Recording Studios with Scrote, Chris
Los Angeles, CA—Credit Christopher Ewing

Later in 2013, when I was ready to stage WADMO, the Universe responded by connecting me with Eron, the artistic director at a local children's theater who was excited about bringing the kids a new experience. In 2015, when I needed to find musical-theater actors to voice the characters but didn't have any connections in the theater world, I put it out into the Universe, and lo and behold, I discovered my casting director and my actors.

When I was raising funds through Kickstarter to release my album, I put my intent and trust in the Universe and surpassed my funding goal. In 2015, I had an idea of creating a pitch video to raise awareness and funds for Cure JM, which would include me, my history with DM, my partnership with Cure JM, and how I use music and art as a healing path. Ten days later, the Universe connected me with Chris, a great local filmmaker, who interviewed me on camera and helped me create my portrait video. What I didn't realize was that creating a pitch video was only scratching the surface. I felt compelled to share my story—my full story of being a singer-songwriter who uses music and art to combat the darkness of DM—and my journey with you in this book in the hope that in turn it might inspire you or give you hope and light in your own times of darkness. When I was ready to write this book and needed an editor experienced with memoirs and health, I found mine. I trust that the Universe gives me exactly what I need at exactly the right time.

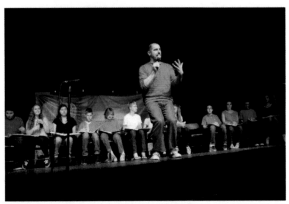

Aoede May 2014 WADMO staged reading with Eron Block
San Carlos Children's Theater, San Carlos, CA—Credit Gregg Harris

Of course, some things I've tried to attract into my life don't transpire in the precise way I imagined, but I stay true to my journey and keep pushing, taking chances, feeling the fear, and doing it anyway despite my disease. I'm still learning to trust my path. When I didn't get a theater residency or grant funding, and a collaboration fell through after a year of trying to produce my third musical, I questioned what the Universe was telling me. Perhaps the message was to find new ways to get at this dream. Perhaps I didn't have the energy or resources to self-produce a full sixteen-show, multiweek production, plus rehearsals, or maybe I wasn't ready. Perhaps I needed time to assemble the right team or find a tech residency.

Little did I know that my next step with *MAGIC* would be to partner with the San Francisco Recreation and Parks Dance and Theater Program to teach ten weeks of original musical-theater workshops. I couldn't have envisioned that the characters, music, and magical world I created in *MAGIC* would inspire fifth and sixth graders, some of whom had never taken part in musical theater before. If I had known that I needed to run workshops, direct staged readings, and further develop the musical to pave the way for a full production with the mentorship of an established theater program in 2017, I would have seen that all the rejections were just the Universe's way of steering me on the right path toward new dreams.

I've learned to trust that if things don't work out the way I envision them, it wasn't the right opportunity or the right path at the time. I choose to remain encouraged, excited by possibility, and not give up hope. My dreams will carry me through anything life throws at me. I use my momentum to keep moving forward. I tell myself I'll find another way. I won't be defeated. I'll keep knocking on doors. I'll continue to believe, persevere, work hard, be creative and passionate, and inspire myself and others on the path to fulfillment and joy. Most important, I'll follow my heart.

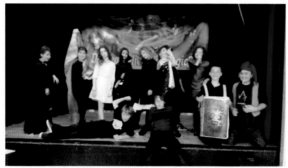

MAGIC cast staged reading Dec 2016,
SF Recreation and Parks, San Francisco

Chapter 11

Being a Light in the Darkness

"Shine. For you are light and wonder. For there are galaxies within you and stardust dances in your soul. Stars live in your eyes, and glory and grace live in your bones. You are beautiful. You are light and wonder. You Shine."

—g.c.

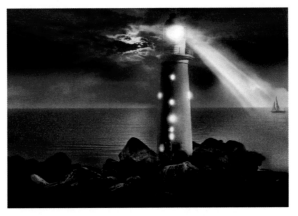

A Light in the Darkness—credit Charlie Aspinall (Chaz Art) 2018

I look back at my darkest days with DM, when I could no longer move my muscles and my life changed in an instant, and I can't help but think about how much support and love enveloped me, how the Universe provided and continues to provide, and how I had everything I needed, inside and out, to get me through.

So many times I asked the Universe, "How I can give back to all of those who have helped and supported me in my time of need?"

The Universe responded, and one message was loud and clear: "Pay it forward."

Early in 2008, as I was researching as much as I could about my new diagnosis, I sought out others who were dealing with DM, discovered online support groups, and connected with my local keep-in-touch group. I also learned of the Myositis Association (TMA) and, later, Cure JM.

In 2011, a year after my hospital stay, just as I was inexplicably compelled to create and share my music, I felt a pressing need to share my story, to use my experience and gifts as a singer-songwriter to help others who were also fighting DM. After being at my lowest point physically and emotionally, I wanted to remind them that their dreams didn't have to die just because they were living with chronic illness.

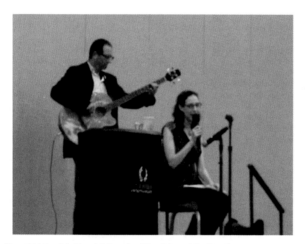

Aoede Sep 2011 with David Sands, The Myositis Conference Las Vegas, NV

I reached out to TMA, explaining that I was a singer-songwriter with DM and was going public with my story in hopes that it would inspire others to pursue their dreams and persevere in spite of myositis. TMA responded by asking me to share my story and perform at their annual conference in September 2011 in Las Vegas. It was an incredible privilege and honor. Though I was still using a wheelchair and walker to get around; relying on David for most of my shopping, cooking, and other basic needs; and dealing with incredible fatigue and lack of stamina anytime I ventured outside the safety and comfort of my house, I felt compelled to go to Las Vegas. It was my way of giving back after all of the support I received during the worst of my illness. Not only was it a milestone of sorts just to deal with the logistics of travel and be present at a multiple-day conference, but it was my first public appearance in more than a year.

I remember when I arrived at the hotel and checked in. All I saw when I looked around were adults, many of whom looked older than I was at thirty-eight. I had mixed feelings. On the one hand, I wasn't ready to see myself with a lifetime of DM ahead of me. On the other hand, here were sixty-five-, seventy-five-, and eighty-year-olds, some in wheelchairs and scooters or using canes, who were managing their illnesses seemingly well—at least well enough to travel and have energy to attend a conference. That encouraged me. I talked to and found common ground with many wonderful people of various ages and stages who shared my disease, and that felt incredibly supportive and empowering. Many of them shared their stories with me, and I learned as much from them as I did from the experts.

After I told my story and sang and played my guitar from my heart, people came up to thank me and tell me what kind of impact I had on them. It made me realize how significant being there was: connecting through story and song with people who understood just what I was going through. It helped me see the kind of inspiration and light in the darkness I could become to the very people who needed it most.

It was at this conference I learned about Cure JM, a group of committed, passionate, driven parents, families, and friends who are successfully raising awareness and funds for kids with the same disease I have. Cure JM recently raised $500K for research, and according to GreatNonprofits, the organization ranks in the top 1 percent of US nonprofits, having raised more than $11 million through grassroots fund-raising! Even though I was older, I somehow identified more closely with the younger adults, perhaps because I've never stopped seeing myself as a kid!

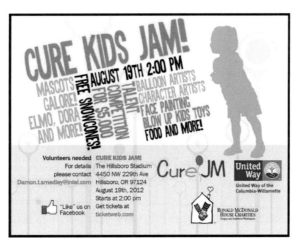

Aug 2012, Cure Kids Jam flyer Hillsboro, OR

In 2012, when I was asked if I was interested in helping Cure JM by telling my story and performing at their festival and fund-raiser in Oregon that summer, I didn't hesitate to accept, despite the toll traveling, performing, and being in the sun took on my body, and the amount of energy I expended doing all those activities. Partnering with Cure JM was one of the tangible ways I could be a light in the darkness to those who needed support during their most difficult times. My hope was that seeing someone who shares their disease tell her story and perform would inspire the kids and give them hope for their own futures.

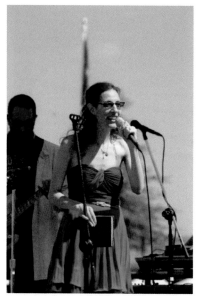

Aoede Aug 2012 with David Sands
Cure Kids Jam and Festival Hillsboro, OR

During my opening remarks at the Cure JM festival, I shared that this wasn't just about being entertained; we were there to share our stories so that we could feel less alone; connect with, support, and inspire one another; and raise awareness and generate more research and funding so that one day cures, not just treatment and symptom management, would be commonplace. We were also there to remember the lights that went before us: tireless fighters and advocates like Mason, the festival coordinator's extraordinary ten-year-old son who was the inspiration for the event. I had never met Mason, who battled JM most of his life. He was a spokesperson for Cure JM and had a profound impact on every life he touched. I intended to meet him at the festival, but he passed away in June of 2012 from JM complications.

His dream was to fill the stadium with free snow cones for all. I had a snow cone in his honor.

After my positive experience at the Cure JM festival, I continued to partner with the organization to help raise awareness and funds by donating proceeds from downloads of my song "Perfect Day" as part of Cure JMs Songs for a Cure fund-raiser. I wrote "Perfect Day" in June 2011 after communicating with a bedridden fan who also suffers from a debilitating muscle disease and is in constant need of breathing support. In spite of his illness, this fan finds empowerment, motivation, and great joy through webmastering a site for an orchestra. He's also passionate about his hobby of ship spotting from his bed and loves to discover, support, and promote new recording artists, like Aoede, on the Internet.

When I first read his story, it brought me to tears. Then my muse immediately started flowing, and out came a new song as I envisioned the world through his lens. After reading his story, I realized it wasn't just his journey I was lamenting; it was my own. It was the first time I let myself acknowledge my own limitations and feel in song what I had been going through.

Perfect Day

I'd feel so alive
I'd feel so alive

Can you see
Can you see me
Do you know
Do you know what I would do
I would do with
Just one perfect day

I would shed
I would shed
My skin this thin veneer
It keeps me here
It keeps me wanting
More than this

I'd feel so alive
I'd feel so alive

Do you see
Do you see me
Can you paint
Can you paint a picture for me
Picture perfect blue sky
Sunny day

Paint the trees
Paint the trees
Apple green make me believe
These leaves are real
Green leaves are falling
One perfect day

I'd feel so alive
I could skip around the sun
Climb a cloud to the moon
I'd feel so alive
On just one perfect day with you

Can you see
Can you see me
Do you know
Do you know what I dream of
I dream of breathing easy
One perfect day

See the ship
See the ship
It glides
And I-I catch a ride
Ride into the sunset
One perfect day

I'd feel so alive
I'd feel so alive

Do you see
Do you see me
Can you show
Can you show me
City life pretty life made easy
One perfect day

Paint the towns
Paint the towns
All around-around me
Set me right beside the nine to fives
One perfect day

I'd feel so alive
I could skip around the sun
Climb a cloud to the moon
I'd feel so alive
I could jump high in the sky
Race a star to the moon

I'd feel so alive
On just one day to dream with
One more day to dance with
Just one perfect day with you[9]

In 2013, I found myself wanting to honor these Cure JM warriors in a special way, so I decided to create a music video for "Perfect Day" that included pictures and drawings from Cure JM kids and even made it into a contest for kids to submit original artwork symbolizing their perfect day. I wanted to give these kids the special gift of seeing themselves as superheroes because that is what they are as they battle the enemy, this god-awful disease and its complications, day in and day out instead of just being … kids.

I researched and found a company that creates a superhero comic generator online and contacted them. Surprisingly, I received a prompt response. After learning what I was trying to do, the principal at HEROized offered to sponsor and create a Cure JM Warrior set for their free superhero generator so the kids could generate their own heroes, which could then be used in my *Perfect Day* video. It worked perfectly! Using pictures of the kids' faces, I transformed them into superheroes and included their special cartoon faces in the video. Years later, Cure JM warriors are still creating their own superheroes with the online generator!

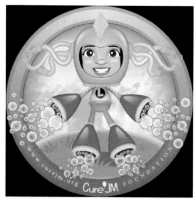

HEROized Cure JM Warrier Set superhero generator
Credit heroized.com

Being a light in the darkness propels me forward in everything I do. Sometimes it's posting an inspirational quote on Facebook or sending out online newsletters to my fans. I've come to see this continual online engagement and positive interaction with others as another way I give back and can be a light. Sometimes it's writing a song and sharing a video that someone's story or a personal event has sparked, such as my song "Perfect Day." Sometimes it's donating to other musicians' and artists' Kickstarter campaigns, going to their concerts, and sharing their projects with my fans to show support. Other times it's just a cheerful personal message letting someone know I'm thinking of him or her, that I care, that I want to help, or simply that I understand. Every once in a while, people send me direct messages like this one, reminding me that I'm making an impact and have a purpose:

I want to thank you for something you don't even realize you did.... Last Monday evening, I was hospitalized for chest pains and heart palpitations, which turned out to be nothing, thankfully. Thank you first for the kind words you posted when I let everyone know what was going on.... The love and light were much appreciated. But that's not all.... I was feeling rather down and unwanted. When I got into the car to go home, I went through my CDs, looking for some music to cheer me up. I found your "Skeletons of the Muse" album and popped it in. I must say, it did cheer me up—a lot. And just at a time I really needed cheering up. So I just wanted to thank you for sharing your talent. Your music is joyful, happy, and smile inducing. Thank you for cheering me up when I needed it most. And thank you for interacting so personally with your fans that I can actually write this little thank-you note. Yesterday, you were my muse.

Helping others who are also battling DM, another illness, or even an unexpected and unwanted life change has been and continues to be an important part of my own recovery. As John O'Donohue said, "May you use this illness as a lantern to illuminate the new qualities that will emerge in you."[10] For me that is very fitting, since living with DM helped me discover my purpose: to be a muse and a light in the darkness.

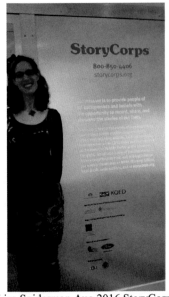

Lisa Sniderman Aug 2016 StoryCorps
San Francisco

In August 2016, David and I had a unique opportunity to record at StoryCorps in San Francisco as part of the Disability Visibility Project (DVP). While talking and reflecting, I had an *aha* moment: I realized that I choose to create light and focus on fantasy, post daily muses, and be so positive to counter the darkness I experience with DM, as well as my rejections and disappointments. Everything I do when I'm living in my place of joy seems to serve my purpose of being a light. I tell stories, connect with others through music and art, and inspire and remind others to love and be filled with gratitude, to wonder, play, create, feel alive, find joy, dream, and never stop believing in magic.

Creating art and music while living with a chronic illness has allowed me to express and continues to help me heal. Through writing my story, I discovered something unexpected: a yearning to be part of something bigger than myself, and a desire to engage and advocate as a disabled artist to encourage and inspire others - especially those experiencing transformations: illness, disability, or unexpected life challenges. Helping you navigate your own personal darkness and heal continues to be an important part of my own recovery. Perhaps I'm only now realizing that DM has been a gift in disguise, and that without this hand I was dealt, I never would have embarked on this journey and discovered my own gifts and true calling. I'm discovering that the most important way I can continue to be a light is to offer my story so that you are inspired to dream, open your heart, and bring to light and share *your* story.

As John O'Donahue would say, may you use it "to illuminate the new qualities that will emerge in you!"

What Makes A Hero

What makes a hero
What makes a hero
Is it super strength or a long cape

What makes a hero
What makes a hero
Am I one today

Does a hero fly (I can fly!)
Is a hero brave (I am bra-a-ave!)
Are there special powers to fight enemies that you can't see … well?

What makes a hero
What makes a hero
Is it spinning webs or secret names

What makes a hero
What makes a hero
Am I one today

Is a hero strong (I am strong!)
Does she save the planet and the day-ay-ay
Does she get knocked down (knocked down)
And get up just to fall-a-gain

What makes a hero
What makes a hero
Is it fighting crime or a bat cave

What makes a hero
What makes a hero
Am I one today

What makes a hero
What makes a hero
Is it never giving up each day

I'll keep on fighting
I'll keep on fighting
This war my body's waged on me again

Oh I'll keep on fighting
I'll keep on fighting
For heroes never stop until they win

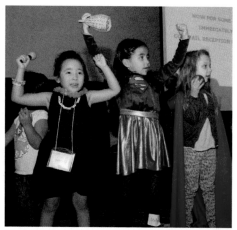

Cure JM Oct 2014 Annual Conference San Jose, CA
Credit Cure JM performing Aoede's "What Makes a Hero"

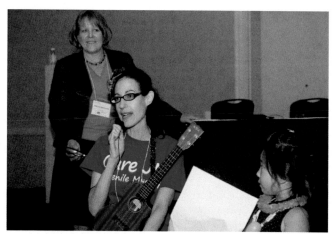

Aoede Oct 2014 Cure JM Conference San Jose, CA

The Hand I Was Dealt

This is the hand
This is the hand I was dealt
This is the hand
This is the hand I was dealt
Guess it's time—oh it's time
I had a good talk with myself

This is the song
I never could write
This is the song
I never wanted to write
But it's time—guess it's time
I laid my cards on the line

Cuz those deep wounds inside
I still cover with smiles
While I wall myself off
From the big world outside
But the dark keeps on calling
Inviting, enticing
I fight it, ignore it
And paint a pretty life but

This is the hand
This is the hand I was dealt
This is the hand
This is the hand I was dealt
And it's time—guess it's time
I stop deceiving myself

This is the place
I never could face
This is the place
I never wanted to face
But it's time—oh it's time
I stop playing it safe

Cuz while everyone tells me
I'm doing so well

I'm pushing so hard
Just to get through this hell
And the dark tries to tempt me
Deplete me, defeat me
I hide it, deny it
And push it aside but

This is the hand
This is the hand I was dealt
This is the hand
This is the hand I was dealt
And I try—oh I try
To feel blessed, see the best in myself

These are the words
That wouldn't come out
These are the words
I needed to come out
And it's time—yes it's time
To say these words out loud

But if I never feel fear
Or the loss or the pain
Then the dark cannot make me
Play its stupid game
But that dark's so alluring,
Enduring, assuring yet
My light is so bright
If I shine it can it cure me

My light
It's so bright
Let it shine
Let it cure me
My light
It's so bright
Let it shine
Let it cure me
My light
Is so bright
Let it shine

Let it cure me

This is the hand
This is the hand I was dealt
This is the hand
This is the hand I was dealt
And it's time—yes it's time
To shine
To shine
To shine

Life Lessons For Living Well With Chronic Illness

* Awaken and greet each day with total love, gratitude and positive attitude
* Keep your spirits high and always have hope
* Strive to get the best quality of life from each day
* Do what you can with what you've got
* Come to peace with a new baseline and slower pace
* Find and live in your place of joy
* Tell yourself and believe you are blessed
* Find and recognize beauty in the little things
* Recognize when you need help; find and embrace a support system in family, friends, and your network
* Don't do this alone! Learn to receive and nurture relationships
* Have empathy and compassion for others
* Make time and opportunity to create and express
* Write about your journey, illness, disability to process, share and connect
* Play, use humor, and find ways to smile and laugh
* Practice the law of attraction: if you imagine it and truly believe it, you can realize it; believe you can attract what is good and positive into your life
* See opportunity from all experiences
* Ask yourself "What can I give?" "What can I learn?" and "What can I teach?" not "Why me?"
* Refuse to be a victim; know you are not the disease
* Be kind to yourself; acknowledge that you will have hard days and better days and listen to your body
* Find community to nurture different passions
* Find ways to give back, share your story, and have impact on others; be a light in the darkness
* Help others who are new to your illness or condition
* Encourage yourself with daily affirmations
* If you aren't able to get out of the house, find and grow an online network
* Find and immerse yourself in something you are passionate about
* Consider making time for creative expression weekly or daily; add to your calendar and make it a habit and practice
* Remember that YOU are enough; where you are and who you are right now is enough

Acknowledgments

I am eternally grateful to my husband, David. Thank you for supporting me during my darkest days with your giving, selfless, loving heart, and for always seeing me and believing in me. You continue to strive and sacrifice every day to provide both of us with the best quality of life and are a true partner in every sense of the word. I attribute so much of my healing to you, your positive attitude, and our love.

Endless gratitude as well to …

My mom and dad, Jan and Lou, for your unconditional support, love, care, sacrifices, and assistance, and for being great role models through my entire illness. Your sincere desire to help and see me heal, and being with me through it all, got me through my hardest times.

My other parents, Florence and Sheldon, for your love, care, support, and encouragement, and for being excellent role models throughout all the stages of my illness. I am so grateful to have you in my life!

My sisters, Helen, Marsha, and Debbie, for being there when I needed support and assistance. Helen, thank you for your visits and for always caring, for being thoughtful and bright, and for our artistic collaborations. Debbie, thank you for taking time out of your life to care for me when I was at my lowest point. Marsha, your calls and concern were always appreciated.

My family and friends, I couldn't have done this without all of you. In particular, thanks to David, Ed, Mark and Jen, Keith, Anna and Thijs, Amy, Jaime, Ruby, Beth, Stacey and Brian, Marianna and Tim, Suzanne, Kristen, Genevieve, Adrienne, Julie and David, Glen and Becky, Florence and Sheldon, Jan and Lou, Helen, and Debbie for your support, for hospital and home visits, and for accompanying me and sitting with me for hours during infusions. Being surrounded by your love and support made all the difference in getting through treatment.

My rheumatologist, Dr. Schwartz, for your excellent care, responsiveness, and concern for more than eight and a half years.

My producer, Scrote, for your years of mentoring; for inspiring me to create, venture outside my comfort zone, and dare to delve into a new artistic niche; for believing in me; and for being my collaborator on multiyear musical-album projects and accommodating me to make it all happen. I wouldn't be where I am today without your amazing vision, attitude, talent, drive, and follow-through.

My Grammy music community, my PR team (particularly Anita and Laura), my mentors Eron and Suze, all the actors and musicians who contributed their talents to my album projects, and all my fans and funders, for your time and dedication, cheerleading, support, promotion, positive reviews, notes and messages, and encouragement despite my health setbacks and rejections.

Mikey Jayy at Artists in Music Awards and Christopher Ewing at Indie Music Channel, for honoring me with my first music awards post-hospital. You pushed me to believe in myself and continue striving for excellence, and you showed me that my music was having an impact.

Joann and Vincent, for sparking the light in me to write this memoir, including my story, Music Is My Lifeline and I Can't Stop Creating, in your book: "88 + Ways Music Can Change Your Life."

My editor, Traci, for your time, efforts, encouragement, and patience, and for pushing me at each step to go further and let my voice come through. I'm so fortunate the Universe put us together, as I couldn't have written this book without your skilled hand helping me craft it! Jennifer, thank you for your incredible eye for detail and skilled fine-tuning instincts.

My publisher, Carly at Crimson Cloak, for believing in me and this book, and for launching me into a world of voice-over work.

The Myositis Association (TMA) and Cure JM Foundation, for being great resources and communities during my early years with DM, and for letting me give back by involving me in your conferences. Shannon and Suzanne, you are amazing, warm-hearted, dedicated parents and organizers, and I'm so glad we've become friends and partners.

Rupam, for your friendship through the years, your generosity, and your kind, warm, selfless heart; and to Chris, for your vision and heart. Thank you both for helping me create the portrait video that accompanies this book.

Ryan, for making all of my musical stories come to life with your vivid, imaginative, detailed illustrations.

Questions For Reflection

1. Have you found a supportive community you can reach out to? Do you feel you're ready to share your story? Who might be inspired by hearing your story?

2. Are you aware of and listening to what your body is telling you? What simple changes could you make to better manage your illness or life?

3. What are your expectations and goals for living with your illness?

4. What are some of the ways you could feel more comfortable with who you are and what you're capable of doing now? What positive messages could you tell yourself to reinforce your strengths, self-confidence, and abilities?

5. Do you feel confident that you've explored your treatment options and are comfortable with your choices as you move forward?

6. What opportunities can you pursue that will enable you to express your creative self and connect more with your friends, family or fans?

7. What inspires or compels you? How can you use this to spark your own creativity? If you're still searching for your passion, what can't you go a day without thinking or dreaming about? What steps can you take now to immerse yourself in some aspect of this dream?

8. What can you do today, this week, and this month to move yourself closer to your dream or creative passion? What could you be doing to challenge yourself and step outside your comfort zone?

9. What resources and program areas could you research and apply for implement to bring you peace of mind, improve your quality of life, or help reduce stress related to your illness or disability (e.g., financial resources, house cleaning, transportation, shopping)?

10. What mini or major milestones have you recently reached on your road to recovery that you can celebrate to lift your spirits?

11. What are some of the ways you can be a light right now, whether championing your own cause or supporting someone else's? What causes are you passionate about that you could use your art to help bring to light?

12. How has fear controlled and limited the way you think and act? What are you doing to tackle that fear?

13. How do you deal with rejection, and what drives you to keep pursuing your dream?

14. What do you turn to when you don't want to focus on your medical issues?

15. How do you define and measure success? Do you find that how you view success changes over time?

16. What makes you feel most alive and connected to others?

17. What does disability mean to you, and do you identify with being disabled? If so, in what way?

18. How can you keep your dreams alive? What are you capable of? What can you continue doing? And if you can no longer do that, what else might you be able to do so that your dream stays alive?

Notes

1. Aoede, "Skeletons," Skeletons of the Muse © 2012 Aoede Muse Music.

2. Margo J. Bendewald, "Incidence of Dermatomyositis and Clinically Amyopathic Dermatomyositis: A Population-based Study in Olmsted County, Minnesota," Archives of Dermatology 146, no. 1 (January 2010):26–30, http://jamanetwork.com/journals/jamadermatology/fullarticle/420951

3. Michelle Lockey Courses, "Fearlessly Alive," accessed April 11, 2017, http://michellelockeycourses.teachable.com/p/fearlessly-alive.

4. See, for example, Heather L. Stuckey and Jeremy Nobel, "The Connection between Art, Healing, and Public Health: A Review of Current Literature," American Journal of Public Health 100, no. 2 February 2010): 254–63, www.ncbi.nlm.nih.gov/pmc/articles/PMC2804629/; Li Qing, "Effect of Forest Bathing Trips on Human Immune Function," Environmental Health and Preventive Medicine 15, no. 1 (January 2010): 9–17, www.ncbi.nlm.nih.gov/pmc/articles/PMC2793341/; Jennifer E. Stellar et al., "Positive Affect and Markers of Inflammation: Discrete Positive Emotions Predict Lower Levels of Inflammatory Cytokines," Emotion 15, no. 2 (April 2015): 129-33, http://dx.doi.org/10.1037/emo0000033.

5. Aoede/Lisa Sniderman, "If You Already Knew," Affair with the Muse © 2011 Aoede Muse Music.

6. Christopher Reeve speech, Democratic National Convention, Chicago, IL, August 26, 1996.

7. Lisa Sniderman, "50 Things I Fell in Love With," © 2009.

8. Robert E. Johnson, quoted in Robert E. Johnson, "Ebony Interview with Mike Tyson," Ebony, September 1995.

9. Aoede/Lisa Sniderman, "Perfect Day," Skeletons of the Muse © 2012 Aoede Muse Music.

10. "A Blessing on the Arrival of Illness," in John O'Donohue, An Abundance of Blessings: 50 Meditations to Illuminate Your Life (London: Bantam Press, 2013).

Resources

CHRONIC ILLNESS

Chronic Illness Awareness Coalition is a coalition of individuals dedicated to improving the quality of life of persons affected with chronic illness, conditions and disabilities. See: http://www.cicmich.org.

HealingWell.com is an online community that provides support and resources (articles, news, videos, message forums, chats) on a wide variety of diseases and health conditions. See: https://www.healingwell.com.

Lights in the Darkness is a virtual support group for passionate artists, musicians and authors who use creativity to help themselves or others heal. It is a place to share the connections between creativity (stories, music, art) and healing. See Facebook Group: Lights in the Darkness: Artists, Authors, Musicians Creating to Heal: https://www.facebook.com/groups/433332727132078/.

MedlinePlus is the National Institutes of Health's website for patients and their families and friends and provides information about diseases, conditions, and wellness issues. For resources for coping with chronic illness, see: https://medlineplus.gov/copingwithchronicillness.html.

The Mighty is a digital health community created to empower and connect people facing health challenges and disabilities. See: https://themighty.com/.

MusiCares is the Recording Academy's charity and provides a safety net of critical assistance, resources and services for music people in times of need that cover a wide range of financial, medical, and personal emergencies. MusiCares also focuses the music industry's resources and attention on human service issues that directly impact the health and welfare of the music community. See: https://www.grammy.com/musicares.

Our Heart Speaks is a resource for individuals living with chronic medical conditions and new disabilities. The site provides an online library and community for individuals to share stories of rehabilitation and healing through personal narrative, poetry, photography, video, artwork and music. See: https://ourheartspeaks.org.

The Spoon Theory is Christine Miserandino's personal story and analogy of what it is like to live with sickness or disability. See: https://butyoudontlooksick.com/articles/written-by-christine/the-spoon-theory/.

Suffering the Silence is a 501(c)3 organization dedicated to leveraging the power of art, media, and storytelling to raise awareness and break the stigma surrounding the life experience of people living with chronic illnesses and disability. See: http://www.sufferingthesilence.com.

"Who Cares: Chronic Illness in America" is a resource list of websites related to chronic care, chronic illness, and disease and includes medical news stories, latest research on various diseases, and online communities. It is based on the topics covered by "Who Cares: Chronic Illness in America," a PBS KQED Television program that aired November 11, 2001. See: https://www.pbs.org/inthebalance/archives/whocares/resources.html.

DERMATOMYOSITIS/MYOSITIS

Cure JM Foundation is a 501(c)(3) nonprofit organization focused on finding a cure and better treatments for the rare and life-threatening autoimmune disease Juvenile Myositis and improving the lives of families affected by JM. See: http://www.curejm.org.

"Keep In Touch" physical support groups and chapters provide members the opportunity to get together with others in their geographic area and share concerns, friendship, and ideas. See: The Myositis Association (TMA), https://www.myositis.org/patient-support/support-groups/ or Cure JM Foundation, http://www.curejm.org/local-chapters/chapter_home.php.

The Myositis Association (TMA)'s mission is to increase support, awareness and funding for the myositis patient, caregiver and research community. The aim of TMA's programs and services is to provide information, support, advocacy, and research for those concerned about myositis. See: https://www.myositis.org.

Virtual Support Groups. Many social media and social networking groups exist online specifically to support people who have myositis. Examples include Facebook groups, such as Myositis "Ramblers" Keep In Touch Group and Cure JM Foundation, and MYO-Connect (for members of TMA), which can provide support where no Keep in Touch groups exist, or for members who are physically unable to attend local meetings. See: https://www.myositis.org/patient-support/support-groups.

Thank you for choosing this book. If you enjoyed it, please consider telling your friends or leaving a review on Goodreads or the site where you bought it. Word of mouth is an author's best friend and much appreciated.

About the Author

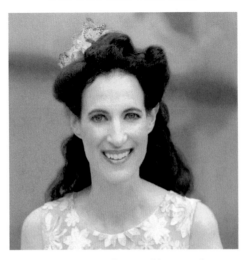

© 2018 Steven Gregory Photography

Award-winning singer-songwriter, artist, playwright, and author Lisa Sniderman, aka Aoede, has garnered numerous accolades for her music and art; engaged fans through social media; participated in national motivational speaking engagements in which she offered support, advice, and encouragement; and received more than fifty awards for her songwriting, audiobooks, and stage plays since 2012.

She's accomplished all of this, and more, in quite an unorthodox fashion and against a very fierce obstacle—a rare, progressive muscle-weakness disease "dermatomyositis" for which there is no known cure. Faced with what, to some, would seem like a battle against insurmountable odds, Sniderman revels in the challenges she faces every day. To listen to Aoede's seven albums, one would never suspect that the individual responsible for this radiant and inspirational body of work continually faces unknown risks and rewards from years of radical and experimental treatments.

While living with a chronic illness, Sniderman creates, records, and shares her original musicals, art, music, and books as a healing path and seeks to be a light and a muse by using her gifts and experience. Says Sniderman, "Music and art are my lifelines, and I just cannot stop creating."

To connect with the author, and for more information, visit …
Aoede at https://alightinthedarkness.info and https://aoedemuse.com
Do You Believe in Magic? at http://doyoubelieveinmagic.info
What Are Dreams Made Of? at http://whataredreamsmadeof.com
Is Love a Fairy Tale? at http://isloveafairytale.com
Aoede Facebook page at http://facebook.com/aoedemusemusic
Aoede Twitter at http://twitter.com/aoedemuse

Also by Lisa Sniderman

Unique, Award-Winning Fantasy Musical-Story Audiobooks!

A meld of Magic, Mythology, and Music!

Colorful characters, compelling stories, infectious songs, danceable duets, narration, sound effects, and full musical score!

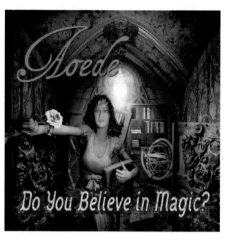

The magical kingdom of Wonderhaven is under a malicious curse. Aoede the Muse believes she has no magic, yet she is the only one who can save the kingdom. (2015)
"Harry Potter and Percy Jackson meet Into The Woods."
(http://doyoubelieveinmagic.info)

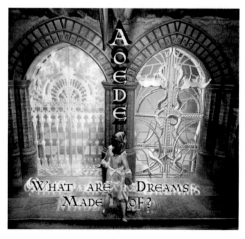

Aoede the Muse is haunted by a nightmare and must confront magical fairies, goblins, and dream gods to get to the heart of her dream. (2013)
"If this album were any better it would be on Broadway!"
(http://whataredreamsmadeof.com)

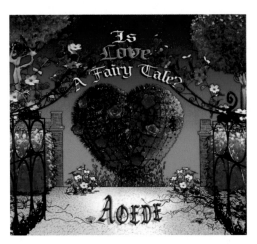

Aoede the Muse searches for love in a magical kingdom called Wonderhaven and meets colorful characters along the way who each tell her something about love. (2012)
"A musical journey that, in the end, leaves one tickled and in awe."
(http://isloveafairytale.com)

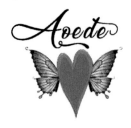

Made in the USA
Monee, IL
19 August 2020